Raw & Simple Detox

First published in the United States of America in 2015 by
Quarry Books, a member of
Quarto Publishing Group USA Inc.
100 Cummings Center
Suite 406-L
Beverly, Massachusetts 01915-6101
Telephone: (978) 282-9590
Fax: (978) 283-2742
www.quarrybooks.com
Visit www.QuarrySPOON.com and help us celebrate food and culture one spoonful at a time!

10 9 8 7 6 5 4 3 2 1

ISBN: 978-1-59253-981-9

Digital edition published in 2015
eISBN: 978-1-62788-162-3

Library of Congress Cataloging-in-Publication Data

Wignall, Judita.
   Raw and simple detox : a delicious body reboot for health, energy, and weight loss / Judita Wignall.
      pages cm
   ISBN 978-1-59253-981-9 (paperback)
1. Raw food diet. 2. Detoxification (Health) I. Title.
   RM237.5.W54 2015
   613.2'65--dc23
                              2014049101

Design: Matt Wignall
Photography: Matt Wignall
Food styling: Peilin Breller

Printed in China

Medical Disclaimer: The following information is intenended for educational purposes only and is in no way intende[...]
Always work with a quailfied health professional before making any changes to your diet. Any application of th[...]
following pages is at the reader's discretions and is his or her sole responsiblity.

Raw & Simple Detox

A Delicious Body Reboot for Health, Energy,
and Weight Loss

Judita Wignall

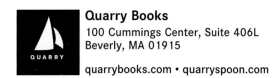

Quarry Books
100 Cummings Center, Suite 406L
Beverly, MA 01915

quarrybooks.com • quarryspoon.com

CONTENTS

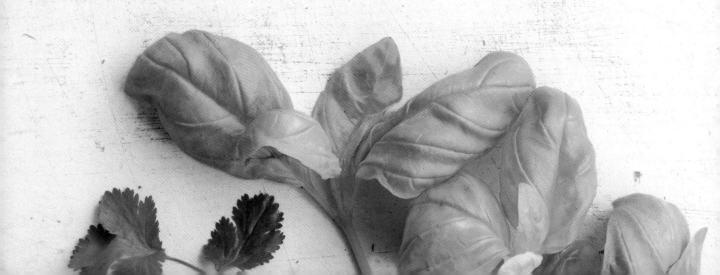

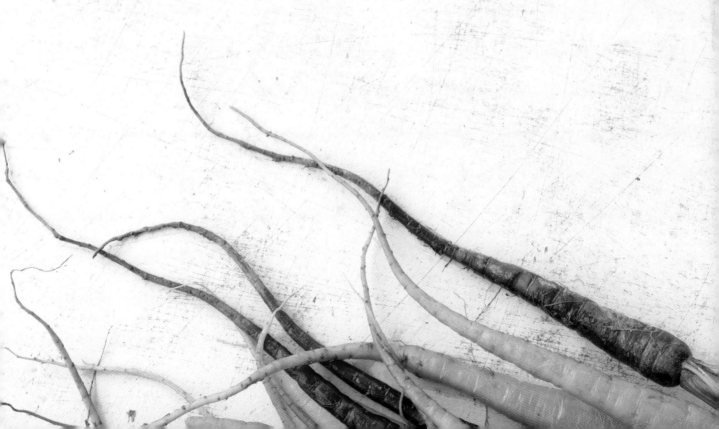

INTRODUCTION

If you haven't already noticed, we live in a very sick world. The Mayo Clinic reported that nearly 70 percent of Americans take at least one prescription drug daily—drugs with side effects that are almost as bad as the symptoms they're created to suppress. About 600,000 Americans die of heart disease every year. About 1,660,000 Americans were diagnosed with cancer in 2013, and about 1,600 people died as a result every day. The adult obesity rate in America is 27.2 percent and rising, and about 347 million people worldwide have diabetes.

We also live in a toxic world. The U.S. Environmental Protection Agency disclosed in its latest report that close to 1 billion pounds of toxic chemicals are introduced into our environment every year through U.S. agriculture alone. I would say that's about 1 billion pounds too many. These chemicals make their way into our municipal water supply, streams, lakes, and oceans, not to mention onto our dinner plates. We also have to deal with air pollution from our cars, coal plants, and other industries.

Chemical manufacturing companies produce 6.5 trillion pounds of 9,000 different chemicals each year; 7 billion pounds of these are released into the atmosphere and water, while 2 billion pounds are recognized carcinogens. On top of that, the Fukushima nuclear plant in Japan continues to melt down and release radioactive particles into the air and ocean. *Science of the Total Environment* journal reported the radioactive plume from that disaster has contaminated the entire Northern Hemisphere and, according to U.S. Nuclear Regulatory Commission records, 75% of American nuclear plants are currently slowly leaking as well. The assault from pollution and our poor diets are putting our health in great danger.

We are literally killing ourselves slowly with toxic chemicals in our food, water, and air. This is not something we can fix with a fad detox kit. If we don't make a conscious effort to live a clean life and lighten the toxic burden on our bodies, we will become a statistic, eventually, as well.

Thankfully, an awakening is happening. Juice bars are popping up all over the country, and the desire to cleanse has never been more popular. People from all walks of life are discovering the benefits of fasting and the power of fresh fruits and vegetables.

My personal awakening happened June of 2007 when I embarked on my first raw food cleanse. I was desperate to get rid of my adult acne, so I jumped in 100 percent. In one month I lost 15 pounds, eliminated the arthritis in my hands, lifted my depression, improved my energy tenfold, and cleared up my skin. I eventually left my career as a commercial actor to become a raw food chef and health coach. Pretty radical for someone who was just experimenting with a new diet!

In addition to eating raw, I've also tried several juice fasts over the years with great results. I have seen friends completely transform from doing long-term juice fasting (also called juice feasting). If you want to see an incredible documentary on how juicing changed the lives of two men, check out *Fat, Sick & Nearly Dead* by Joe Cross.

Though I love the juice detox model, it can be too extreme for some. In this book, I want to introduce a way for people to get the benefits of juice fasting while still maintaining a somewhat regular diet. I don't know about you, but I love to eat—and the great news is, you can still eat delicious food while helping your body to cleanse and reset.

The first step of this plan is to eliminate the foods and toxic chemicals that cause disease. Second, we want to give your digestion a rest while flooding your body with vitamins, minerals, antioxidants, and immune-boosting, age-defying phytonutrients. Whether you just need a day or so to detox from an overindulgent holiday or a monthlong body reset, this book contains easy recipes to help up your energy and get you looking and feeling your best.

I want to preface that this is not a weight-loss guide. But if you're carrying around excess waste in your colon and retaining water, you should see that extra baggage come right off, and then some. Doing a detox is a great way to start a weight-loss program, as sometimes our body is resistant to letting go simply because it's so toxic. Let the weight loss be a bonus and focus on eating high-quality, nutrient-dense foods. Learn new ways to incorporate these detox principles into your daily life where, every day, you can help your body more efficiently do what it does naturally.

Use this book as a springboard to go into whatever diet works for you. Whether you want to continue on a raw journey, go paleo, or anywhere in between, this is a great way to clean out your system before you rebuild using whatever foods work best for you.

Please keep in mind that I'm a healthy-lifestyle coach and whole foods chef, not a doctor. All the information described in this book is for educational purposes only and not meant to treat any medical condition. If you have any chronic health issues, consult your doctor first. If you are underweight, have very low energy, or have any weakness, a cleanse is not recommended. Please use good judgment as you apply the principles in this book.

This can be a very powerful and health transforming journey. I hope you enjoy the experience and discover vibrant health like you've never had before.

Happy cleansing!

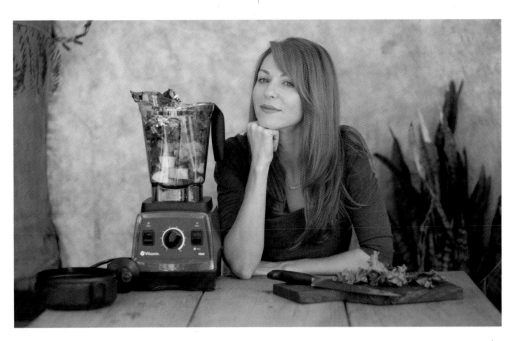

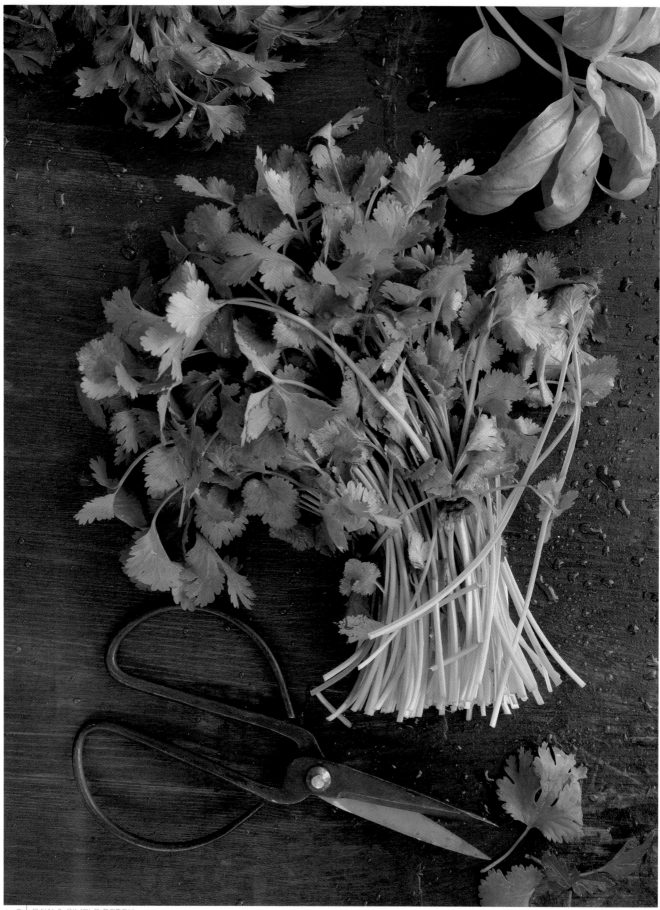

CHAPTER 1

WHAT IS A RAW DETOX?

Detoxification simply means to remove toxins—the environmental and man-made chemicals that accumulate in our body over time through our modern lifestyle. Our bodies are self-healing and will take care of foreign matter as needed all day long, but there can still be an overload as more toxins than we can eliminate enter the body. It's an unfortunate reality of our chemical-filled world. This overload results in reduced energy and organ function, inflammation, nutritional deficiency, accelerated aging, and disease. There are many methods and opinions on how to move the junk out, but the way that I've helped my clients do this gently and with the least amount of side effects is to eat your way to health with raw foods like fresh fruits, vegetables, avocados, coconuts, nuts, and seeds.

A raw food diet consists of eating foods that have not been heated over 118°F (48°C), thereby preserving their full nutritional content. At 118°F (48°C), we start to break down the enzymes, and at 135°F (57°C), we begin to lose the vitamins and phytonutrients in the food. A typical cooked meal only has around 50 to 70 percent of the nutrients it had before it was heated. No heat means that the carbohydrates (sugars) haven't caramelized, fats are not adulterated and sticky, and the protein amino acid chains are intact and bioavailable. Every raw meal gives you more bang for your buck, nutritionally speaking, and is packaged in the way Mother Nature intended for us, not stripped, processed, and refortified, with added preservatives and artificial chemicals like most of the food on grocery store shelves today.

Besides eating more nutrient-dense meals, we're also lightening up the digestive load. It takes a lot of energy to digest food from our stomach to, well, the finish line. Our digestive tract is 20 to 30 feet (6 to 9 m) long and involves several major organs, such as the esophagus, stomach, small and large intestines, pancreas, liver, and gallbladder. In this plan, we'll be enjoying lots of easy-to-digest foods like juices, smoothies, and soups. Eating light gives our body more energy to work on removing toxins and repairing tissues and cellular function; in

short, we are supporting the natural cleansing process of the body. Other great benefits to raw food are that it also contains fiber to help sweep out waste in the digestive system and water to hydrate the colon and tissues. Having great digestion is the heart of great health, as you'll see later on in this book.

Because raw foods are so high in antioxidants, they are anti-inflammatory foods. Inflammation is an immune response that occurs when cells are signaled to respond to an injury or foreign stimuli like carcinogens, toxins, fungi, or pathogens. This is the body's way of protecting itself and is an important part of healing. When inflammation is coming from a toxic environment or diet, eating antioxidant-rich raw foods can help neutralize free radicals that cause damage within the body, like in the arteries (such as plaque), joints (such as arthritis), and eyes (such as macular degeneration). So consider this an anti-inflammatory diet as well as a detox and a major step in slowing degenerative disease.

But the power of a raw food detox lies not in just what we eat, but also what we don't eat. Let's face it. The Standard American Diet (SAD . . . sad indeed) is quite toxic.

IN THIS DETOX WE OMIT:

- Processed foods that have been stripped of nutrients
- Industrial seed oils that are rancid and inflammatory
- High-fructose corn syrup that is linked to obesity, diabetes, and fatty liver disease
- Artificial sweeteners that are neurotoxins
- Trans fats that cause inflammation and heart disease
- MSG, which is a neurotoxin and linked to diabetes
- Artificial flavors, colors, and preservatives that are neurotoxins
- Genetically modified foods that cause tumors in lab rats and are linked to liver failure and infertility

OUR MODERN TOXIC LIFE

So what exactly are these toxins? Toxins can be heavy metals like mercury from our dental amalgams, aluminum from our cookware, or cadmium from cigarettes and fertilizer. It can be halogens like chlorine from tap water, fluoride from toothpaste, or bromine from bread. It could be pesticides, herbicides, and fungicides from farming. They can be chemicals that are in our water, cosmetics, prescription medication, and furniture. They can be the byproduct of factories and automobiles. There is almost no man-made thing that doesn't contain some sort of chemical that is harmful to our health.

And try as we may, we will never be toxin free. Our world is so polluted, we will never return to a point where we have pristine water, air, or soil ever again. And there is no detox that can remove all toxins forever. Fortunately, our bodies are resilient and adaptable. Even as babies today are born with an average of 287 man-made chemicals in their umbilical cords, according to the Environmental Working Group, they can still thrive in a toxic world. The goal of this book is not to be rid of toxins, but to help our body function better so it can handle the daily exposure.

HOW DO YOU KNOW IF YOU'RE TOXIC?
Here are a few signs from your body that something is out of balance:

- Acne
- Bloating
- Gas
- Constipation
- Diarrhea
- Recurring infections
- Depression
- Anxiety
- Mood swings
- Hormonal imbalance
- Headaches
- Fatigue
- Arthritis
- Inflammation
- Muscle weakness
- Allergies
- Sinus infections
- Asthma
- Sore throat
- Brain fog
- Rashes
- Eczema
- Infertility

These are signals that we need to pay attention to our body. Don't ignore these symptoms or suppress them with pills. If you address the source of the problem, you can get rid of them for good. If your car engine is making noise, you don't just turn the radio up louder. You fix the problem.

HOW WE STORE AND RELEASE TOXINS
The major organs involved in the detoxification process are the liver, small intestines, kidneys, and lymphatic system, while the exit doors are our large intestine, lungs, bladder, and skin. All of them are important in the detoxification process, but the organs we'll focus on mainly in this book are the liver and the small and large intestines.

Our liver is the filter and cleanser of the blood and the major detoxifier of the body. It has two major detoxification phases when toxins enter the body. Phase one is called oxidation. In this phase, the liver uses oxygen and enzymes to make the toxins water soluble, while in phase two, called conjugation, the oxidized compounds are combined with sulfur, specific amino acids, and organic acids before being excreted in the bile.

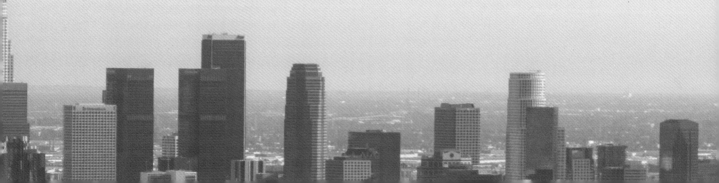

It's very important that both phases are working properly and that enough nutrients are available, especially in phase two, in order to allow detoxification to happen efficiently. For many people, phase one is overactive and phase two is sluggish. By supporting both phases at the same time, we can have an efficient liver and avoid detox side effects.

FOODS AND SUPPLEMENTS THAT SUPPORT PHASE ONE PATHWAYS ARE:

- Cruciferous vegetables, such as cabbage, broccoli, and brussels sprouts
- Curcumin from turmeric
- Antioxidants and folate from raw fruits and vegetables
- Citrus fruit, especially grapefruit juice

FOODS AND SUPPLEMENTS THAT SUPPORT PHASE TWO PATHWAYS ARE:

- Alliums and sulfur from garlic, onions, and scallions
- Bioflavanoids from citrus fruit and vegetables such as peppers, celery, and carrots
- Curcumin from turmeric
- Sulfur from cruciferous vegetables
- Betalain from beets
- Sylimarin from milk thistle
- Flaxseed oil
- Liposomal glutathione
- Chlorella
- Cilantro
- Methylsulfonylmethane (MSM)

When the liver becomes overburdened and cannot eliminate them fast enough, toxins enter the bloodstream. Many of the toxins and heavy metals in our bodies are fat-soluble. That means they are attracted to and dissolve in fats and oils, such as our adipose tissue (body fat) as well as the brain, breasts, thyroid, and cell membranes. Here they stay until released by dieting, exercising, stress, or sweating. Their release can sometimes be accompanied by headaches, fatigue, brain fog, nausea, or general malaise. For someone who lives a sedentary life, these toxins can be stored indefinitely. Unfortunately, even fat cells have a limit to how many toxins they can handle. When they become oversaturated, toxins are again released into the bloodstream, where they eventually settle into more available cells.

Having overburdened fat cells is one reason why some people cannot lose weight. They diet, even eating much less than a thin person, yet the weight doesn't budge. That's because they can't override the body's protective function, which is to stow away the toxins. This is why a detox is a great way to kick off a weight-loss diet plan.

Besides supporting our liver, we also need to focus on our small and large intestines. After our mouths and stomach have done the chewing and have broken down our food into a yummy mixture called chime, the small intestine's job is to extract and absorb the nutrients for our body to use. The large intestine, also known as the colon, then takes the indigestible food matter and scoots it all out. You may be surprised to learn that much of our immune system is dependent on our gut health. If we don't have the right amount of good flora, fiber, and water, and we're loading it up with toxins and excess sugars, things can get pretty complicated in there and lead to a whole array of health issues.

DIGESTION:
THE BASIS OF GOOD HEALTH

Almost all good and bad health leads back to the digestive system. When things are running suboptimally, we can often trace it to an issue somewhere along the digestive process. How is that, you wonder? Well, first let's look at the incredible things that take place in our gut:

▶ About 80 percent of our immune system, the gut-associated lymphatic tissue, or GALT, is found in the digestive system. Immune cells like antibodies, T cells, B cells, mast cells, and phagocytes circulate around the body, but they originate from our gut. We can keep the GALT strong by taking probiotics and eating a good clean diet.

▶ Ever get a "gut feeling" about something? The gut is actually our second brain, also called the enteric nervous system. Researchers have discovered that biochemical signaling takes place between the GI tract and the nervous system in our brain via our intestinal microbiota. In fact, 90 percent of the neurotransmitter serotonin, the one responsible for the feeling of happiness and well-being, is created by the neurons in our gut. There is evidence that some depression and anxiety sufferers may find relief with a gut-balancing and stress-management protocol.

▶ The intestinal flora is our second liver, eliminating 40 percent of the toxins in the food we eat.

When gut function is impaired by processed foods, excess sugar, medications, chlorinated water, antibiotics, stress, or high exposure to toxins, we can develop constipation, leaky gut syndrome, food sensitivities, autoimmune and inflammatory bowel conditions, and hormonal imbalance. Our first line of defense is our microflora.

COCONUT YOGURT:
This is a tasty way to protect your gut. See the recipe on page 168.

BENEFICIAL BACTERIA

We have around 100 trillion bacteria living in our gut. The role of these bacteria is to digest food into small nutrients that we can use. We are only as healthy as what we can absorb, though. If opportunistic organisms take over, we can create nutrient deficiencies and weakened intestinal walls, preventing us from creating neurotransmitters and hormones and compromising our entire immune system. Our gut bacteria are an integrated part of the body and are influenced by our diet and lifestyle. If our internal garden of beneficial bacteria are overtaken by yeast (candidiasis), fungus, parasites, and bad bacteria, we can tip the scales back by taking probiotics in the morning or before bed on an empty stomach and eating fermented foods and beverages with meals. Most of us have some level of dysbiosis of the gut like:

- Gas
- Bloating
- Cramping
- Constipation
- Intense food cravings
- Brain fog

If you are suffering from these symptoms on a daily basis, you may need to cut out fruit and all sugar and carbohydrates from your diet for 6 to 12 weeks, depending how severe it is. Sugar is fertilizer for pathogenic bacteria, yeast, and fungi. I have many fruit/sugar-free options in this book, and you can always use stevia and xylitol to sweeten beverages and chocolate treats if desired.

SIMPLE CLEANSING TIP:

Fermented foods are great detoxifiers, pulling pesticides and chelating heavy metals from our gut. A small serving (¼ cup or 45 g) of cultured vegetables contains much more beneficial bacteria than a probiotic pill alone. You can buy delicious fermented foods from the health food stores. Just make sure it's actually cultured and not pickled in vinegar. You can also make your own Beet Kvass (page 69) on the cheap and enjoy it with meals.

LEAKY GUT SYNDROME

Leaky gut syndrome is terminology used to describe permeable intestines. When the intestinal lining becomes porous, undigested food molecules, yeast, pathogens, toxins, and other types of waste can flow freely into the bloodstream. This can cause diarrhea, chronic constipation, food allergies, inflammatory bowel disease, autoimmune disease like Hashimoto's thyroiditis, rheumatoid arthritis, celiac disease, rosacea, multiple sclerosis, and lupus, impaired immune function, nutritional deficiency, skin conditions like eczema and acne, as well as headaches, fatigue, and brain fog.

SOME CONTRIBUTING FACTORS INCLUDE:

▶ Poor diet. Genetically modified and chemically laden processed foods full of trans fats, refined sugar, preservatives, and artificial colorings can create inflammation in the gut and throughout the body.

▶ Candida. This yeast thrives off sugar. When it gets out of hand, it grows tentacles that burrow into the intestinal lining, perforating it and allowing matter to get through.

▶ Wheat gluten. It's not only people who suffer from celiac disease who need to avoid gluten. Gut inflammation occurs in about 80 percent of the population due to the proteins gliadin and glutenin, which cause intestinal cells to die prematurely. These proteins are found in wheat, semolina, spelt, Kamut, rye, and barley. Some cultivars of oats and quinoa can also create a gut inflammation. (I know, I know. I can practically hear your hearts breaking right now.)

▶ Medication. Medicines like aspirin and acetaminophen decrease the mucosal lining of the intestines.

HEALTH TIP:

If you suspect you have leaky gut, try adding L-glutamine, digestive enzymes, vitamin D_3, zinc, and a good-quality fish oil, along with probiotics and dietary and lifestyle changes to your daily regimen to help restore gut integrity. I recommend the book **Clean Gut** *by Dr. Alejandro Junger for a more in-depth look on how to heal the gut.*

CONSTIPATION

When I tell my coaching clients that they should be eliminating two to three times a day, I get a lot of raised eyebrows. Most people are lucky if they go once a day or every other day, but ideally we should go after every meal. It's crucial for the body to process and eliminate ingested food on a timely basis. Optimal transit time is about twelve to twenty-four hours, but a sluggish bowel could take days in some cases. The average transit time in the Western world is forty-eight to ninety-six hours, with $140 million a year spent on over-the-counter laxatives! Food that is still in the intestinal system after twenty-four hours will start to rot and release toxic substances into the bloodstream. Slow bowels can be caused by poor diet, lack of fiber, dehydration, lack of exercise, stress, travel, candida overgrowth, antibiotics, dairy, medications, leaky gut syndrome, irritable bowel syndrome, diabetes, adrenal fatigue, autoimmune disease, hypothyroidism, or underlying disease.

It's imperative that you get the bowels moving before you start your raw cleanse. Your liver will be releasing toxins that will end up sitting in the intestines and will eventually recirculate in the bloodstream if you're chronically constipated. This can cause fatigue, brain fog, nausea, and mood swings. If you have leaky gut, this can exasperate skin and autoimmune conditions. If you're not eliminating after each meal or you aren't having one substantial movement per day, then implement my constipation remedies on the next page. Once this pathway is clear and functioning, you can start your cleanse.

HEALTH NOTE:

If you still have symptoms of dysbiosis after removing sugars, gluten, and adding in probiotics, you may have small intestinal bacterial overgrowth, or SIBO. You may want to explore the Gut and Psychology Syndrome Diet (GAPS) or the Specific Carbohydrate Diet to balance your gut microbiome and heal the gut lining.

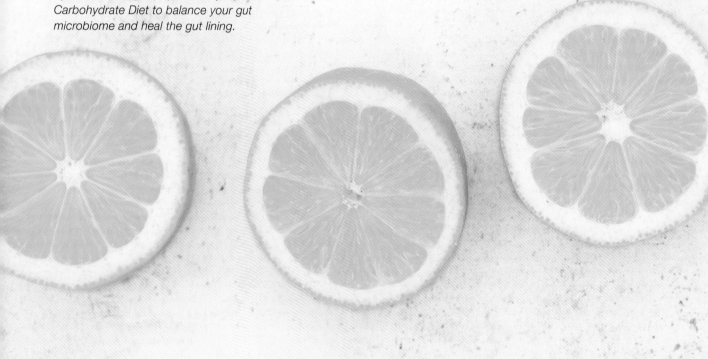

HOW TO ALLEVIATE CONSTIPATION:

- Drink more water. Hot Lemon Water (page 75) in the morning is very helpful to induce peristalsis.
- Eat fiber-rich foods like fruits, vegetables, and especially dark leafy greens.
- Exercise. Yoga stretches are great for waking up the internal organs, while cardio and weights will help speed up your metabolism.
- Ingest probiotics and fermented foods and beverages like sauerkraut, kimchi, kefir, and kvass. Take probiotics first thing in the morning or last thing at night on an empty stomach or have a serving of a fermented beverage like coconut kefir or Beet Kvass (page 69). Sauerkraut and kimchi are great to have with meals.
- Position yourself correctly when you're on the toilet. Squatting is actually the best position for great elimination. You can purchase a footstool called the Squatty Potty or just raise up your toes to get into a semisquat. I've heard some people will actually climb up on the seat, but I'm going to leave that decision up to you.
- Take magnesium citrate before bed. My favorite brand is Natural Calm.
- Take Oxy-Powder or Oxy-Mag. These products use magnesium oxide to oxygenate the entire intestinal tract and pull water in. You will get very watery stool that is the equivalent of having a mild colonic along with adding quite a spring in your step when you're done. Most people tolerate it well, but I recommend starting at the lowest dose and staying near a restroom.
- Have an enema or colon hydrotherapy (page 31).
- Use castor oil. Try 1 teaspoon on an empty stomach before bed or upon rising. Increase the dosage if needed, but do not take it for more than seven days.
- Use herbal and over-the-counter laxatives as a last resort. I don't recommend it because they can irritate or damage the gut, cause severe cramping, and result in your body becoming reliant on them.

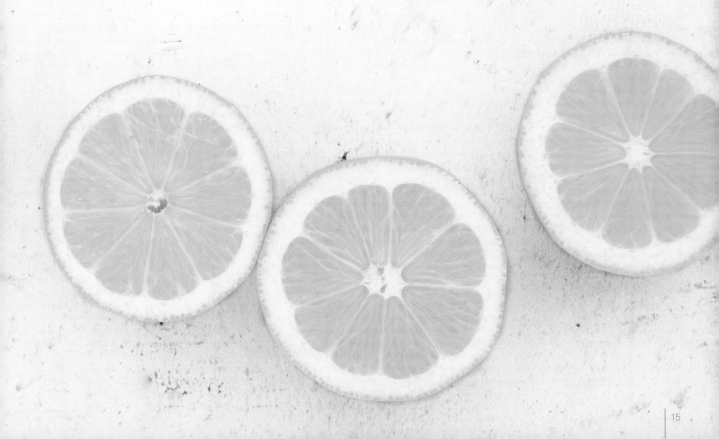

THE RAW & SIMPLE DETOX PROTOCOL

Now that you're familiar with the two major components of cleansing and great health, let's talk about our basic detox protocol, which will be as follows:

1. Decrease toxin exposure in the diet, home, and daily life.

2. Help the body to cleanse naturally with a nourishing raw diet.

3. Assist the liver and the gut in detoxification.

Step one is really the foundation. There is no point of going through the trouble of a detox if you do nothing to clean up your surroundings. Though we can't escape all the toxic chemicals in our world, we certainly have control over how much we come into contact with in our homes.

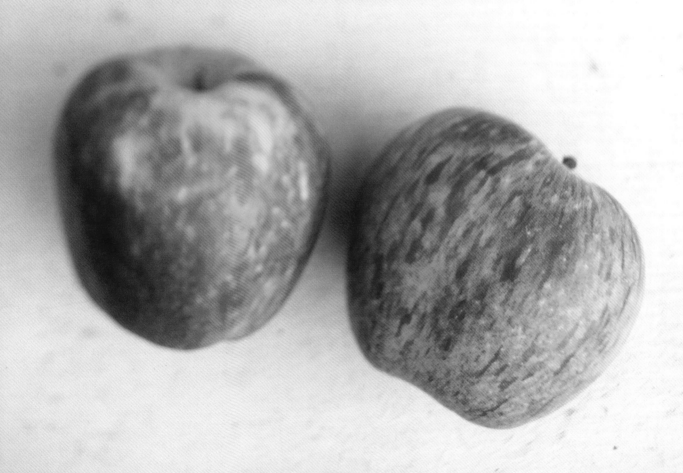

REDUCING TOXIN EXPOSURE AT HOME

By following these clean living tips, you will not only be reducing your toxin exposure dramatically, but also making the world a less polluted place.

1. Buy nontoxic household cleaners and clothing detergent and do not store any chemicals inside your home. The detergent you use to wash your bed sheets and clothing is very important because it never fully rinses from the fabric. Many of these, even so-called eco/natural detergents, contain endocrine disruptors and can create hormonal imbalances like estrogen dominance. The only brand I use is Nature Clean powdered detergent or powdered zeolites. I also recommend tossing out your dryer sheets and using ½ cup (120 ml) of white vinegar in the rinse cycle instead.

2. Get a water filter for your drinking water and shower. A whole house filter would be ideal, but decent systems could cost well over a thousand dollars. Get a good one for the kitchen to wash produce and have drinking water and put a shower filter in your bathroom. Taking a hot, steamy chlorine or chloramine shower is one of the most toxic things you can do in your home. You're basically putting yourself into a low-intensity gas chamber every time you shower. Breathing toxins is more dangerous than ingesting them, as they can enter your bloodstream directly from the lungs.

3. Buy nontoxic cosmetics and personal products. This is especially important with lipstick that you will eventually eat off and deodorant that contains chemicals that absorb into breast tissue and lymph nodes. Remember, the skin will absorb anything you put on it, from moisturizers to tattoos, so be smart with products and be good to your body. My rule of thumb is if you can't eat it, don't put it on your skin. Check out the Environmental Working Group's Skin Deep Database (www.ewg.com/skindeep) to see how toxic your beauty products are. You will be shocked to find how many "natural" products are not so natural. Even better, you can learn how to make your own personal care products with the book *The Home Apothecary* by Stacey Dugliss-Wesselman.

4. Eat organic as much as possible. Keep it within your budget by buying produce that is in season and check out your local farmers' market for great deals and the freshest food. Also check out the Dirty Dozen from the Environmental Working Group (www.ewg.org) to see which pesticide-laden foods are to be avoided at all costs and which conventionally grown food is clean.

5. Get an air filter. Off-gassing from furniture, mattresses, carpets, curtains, and paint can make the air in your home worse than urban city air. We keep a filter in our bedroom at all times and have plants in the rest of the house. Plants are wonderful air filters and transform your room into a true living space. Check out the book *How to Grow Fresh Air* by B. C. Wolverton to learn how to get started.

6. Avoid plastic. Plastic is notorious for containing bisphenol A (BPA), an endocrine disruptor that mimics estrogen in the body. It has been linked to infertility and hormonal imbalance in women and men. A Centers for Disease Control and Prevention study found that 95 percent of adult human urine samples and 93 percent of samples in children contained BPA. Some companies are replacing BPA with bisphenol B, but there is concern that it could actually be even worse than BPA. It's best to just avoid plastics in general as much as possible. Use a glass or metal water bottle (filled with your delicious filtered water from home or spring water if you have any where you live), avoid buying food in plastic packaging, and use glass containers when storing leftovers.

7. Replace your cookware. Teflon-coated cookware can leach toxins into your food, while stainless steel could leach nickel. The best cookware is ceramic or glass made in the USA. Luckily, you won't have to worry about that too much while you're on this cleanse.

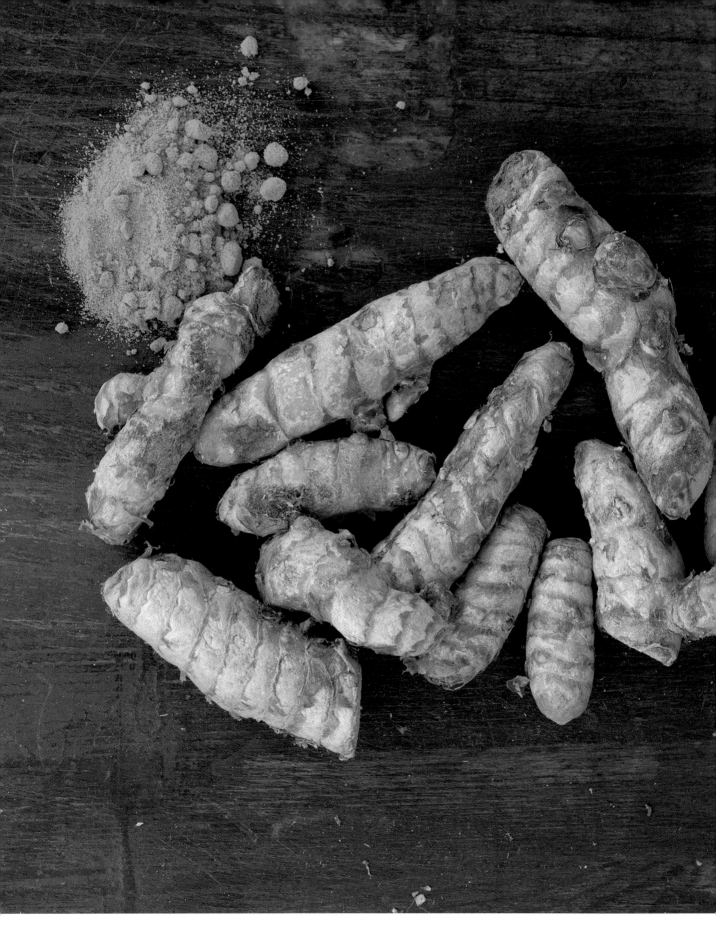

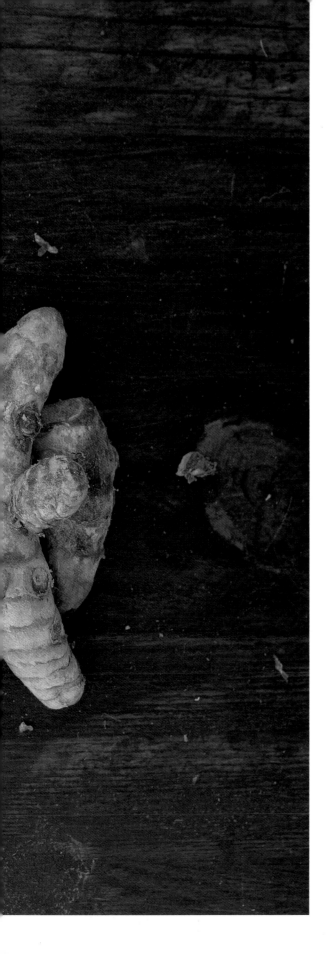

CHAPTER 2

PREPARING FOR SUCCESS

STOCKING THE KITCHEN

Watch your kitchen transform into the garden of Eden as you embark on this cleanse. I love staring at all the gorgeous fresh fruits and vegetables that fill my kitchen. The colors of plump, ripe fruits and vegetables and the fragrance of fresh herbs and seasonings make me feel like a queen. Here are some of the wonderful ingredients you'll be enjoying on this cleanse.

Fruits: lemons, limes, oranges, grapefruit, watermelon, strawberries, raspberries, cranberries, blueberries, banana, pineapple, mango, papaya, apples, pears, grapes, and dried fruits

Vegetables: cucumbers, celery, bell peppers, tomatoes, spinach, zucchini, beets, carrots, romaine lettuce, Swiss chard, cabbage, arugula, watercress, dandelion, kale, onions, sprouts, and burdock root

Good fats: coconuts, avocado, hemp seeds, chia seeds, raw almonds, walnuts, pecans, cashews, and pine nuts, flaxseeds, sesame seeds, pumpkin seeds, sunflower seeds, coconut oil, olive oil, and flaxseed oil

Herbs: basil, parsley, cilantro, mint, scallions, garlic, shallots, ginger, and turmeric root

Seasonings and sweeteners: sea salt/pink salt, vanilla, cayenne pepper, chipotle pepper, coconut aminos, turmeric, curry powder, cinnamon, apple cider vinegar (such as Bragg), raw honey, coconut nectar, liquid stevia, and xylitol granules

SIMPLE CLEANSING TIP:

Starting a new diet can sometimes be overwhelming, but if you get your kitchen in order with the right tools and ingredients, you will make it easier to stick to the plan and ensure your success.

SPECIALTY INGREDIENTS

There are a few items that you may not be familiar with, but you can find them at most health food stores or online. My website carries some of the more unique items. Look for the following:

VANILLA POWDER

This is simply ground vanilla beans. This is less expensive than buying single beans and my preferred way of adding aromatic vanilla to my recipes. If you can't find it, you may also use vanilla extract or flavoring. Extracts are a little more potent while flavorings are sweeter and may require a bit more than extracts in recipes.

SALT

I prefer to use Celtic sea salt, but Himalayan pink salt is also a wonderful choice, as well as many of the artisanal salts available on the market these days. Avoid processed iodized table salt like the plague. I carry a little wooden salt shaker in my purse so I never have to use the cheap salt at restaurants.

STEVIA

I use this zero-glycemic sweetener in the liquid form for many of my beverages, smoothies, and desserts. The best brand is Omica Organics. It has no bitterness and is more potent than store-bought liquid stevia. I do not specify how much to use in recipes, as the intensity will vary between brands. Follow this rule of thumb with stevia: Less is more.

XYLITOL GRANULES

This is also zero glycemic and an alternative to stevia. It's slightly less sweet than sugar. Make sure yours comes from birch trees, not corn, which is usually genetically modified. If you don't care for xylitol, you could also use erythritol or Lakanto, which is made from plant sugars. It is less sweet than xylitol, so you'll need to use a tad more.

COCONUT AMINOS

This is a soy sauce alternative made from coconut sap. It's gluten free, soy free, and raw. I use the Coconut Secret brand. If you can't find it anywhere, you could use wheat-free tamari instead, but it isn't appropriate if you're avoiding soy.

LECITHIN GRANULES

This is an emulsifier used in the food industry for things like chocolate bars, baked goods, and confections. In the raw food world, we like it in desserts and smoothies to keep things from separating, but it is also a wonderful supplement. It's high in the B vitamins choline and inositol, which are great for cognitive repair, eye health, cardiovascular function, skin, and hair. Look for lecithin granules or powder made from sunflower seeds instead of soybeans. If you can only find soy lecithin, use the powder form instead of granules, which contain soybean oil.

COCONUT NECTAR

This is an agave nectar alternative that is lower in fructose and higher in glucose, which is a better sugar for the body to utilize. It has a wonderful caramel-like flavor and texture, and has a lower glycemic index than other natural sweeteners such as honey and maple syrup.

BRAGG APPLE CIDER VINEGAR

This is superior to regular old apple cider vinegar. Bragg is raw, organic, unpasteurized vinegar that is rich in enzymes and beneficial bacteria. It's a wonderful digestive aid and can even be added to your Lemon Water (page 75) for a potent detox drink.

DULSE

This Atlantic Coast seaweed is my preferred sea vegetable. It can be eaten as is straight from the bag and is quite delicious. It's not fishy or overpowering like other seaweeds, but it is still packed with minerals like iodine, manganese, iron, vitamin K, and other trace minerals. You can add it to any salad, soup, or savory smoothie. Buy it in strips or flakes.

KOMBU

Another great sea vegetable to add to your diet, kombu is naturally high in iodine and is a delicious flavoring for soups. I prefer to source the Atlantic over the Pacific variety due to possible radioactive contamination.

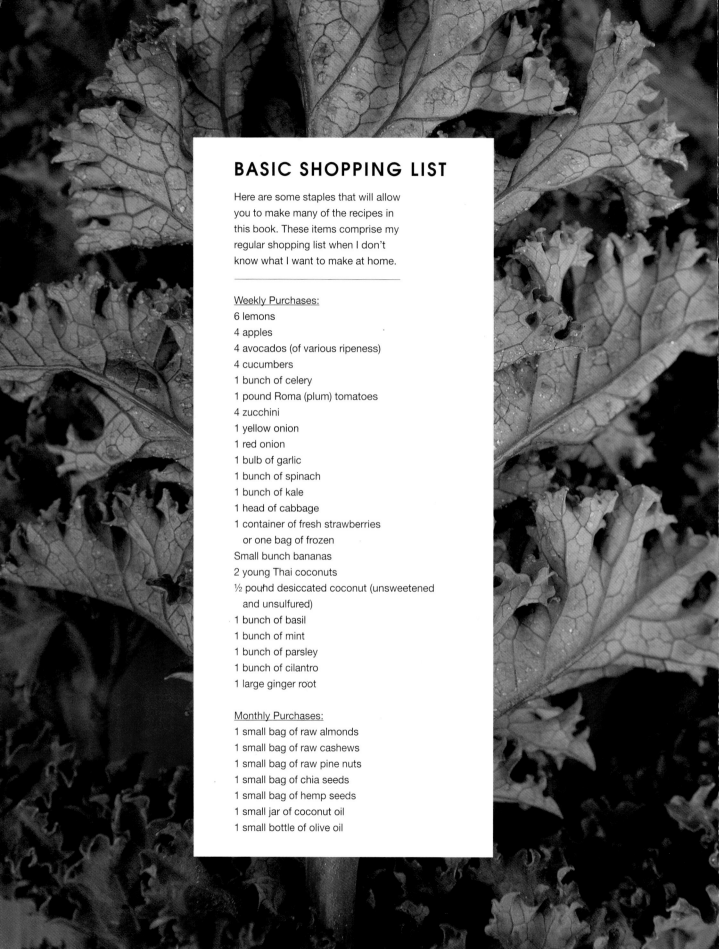

BASIC SHOPPING LIST

Here are some staples that will allow you to make many of the recipes in this book. These items comprise my regular shopping list when I don't know what I want to make at home.

Weekly Purchases:
6 lemons
4 apples
4 avocados (of various ripeness)
4 cucumbers
1 bunch of celery
1 pound Roma (plum) tomatoes
4 zucchini
1 yellow onion
1 red onion
1 bulb of garlic
1 bunch of spinach
1 bunch of kale
1 head of cabbage
1 container of fresh strawberries
   or one bag of frozen
Small bunch bananas
2 young Thai coconuts
½ pound desiccated coconut (unsweetened
   and unsulfured)
1 bunch of basil
1 bunch of mint
1 bunch of parsley
1 bunch of cilantro
1 large ginger root

Monthly Purchases:
1 small bag of raw almonds
1 small bag of raw cashews
1 small bag of raw pine nuts
1 small bag of chia seeds
1 small bag of hemp seeds
1 small jar of coconut oil
1 small bottle of olive oil

PRODUCE TIPS

- Buy organic as much as possible. I know I mentioned organics earlier, but it's worth repeating: Buy organic! If you want to know how pesticides, fungicides, and herbicides affect human health, you simply have to look at the health of workers at conventional farms. The U.S. Environmental Protection Agency estimates that 10,000 to 20,000 farmworkers are poisoned on the job due to pesticide exposure every year. These workers suffer from short-term symptoms such as nausea, vomiting, skin rashes, blisters, and muscle cramps and from long-term problems such as infertility, birth defects, blindness, leukemia, cancer, neurological disorders, and nerve damage. The more we purchase organic produce, the more we support good farming practices, protecting workers and protecting the planet. On the other hand, I understand that some parts of the world don't have much to offer in organics or they're very expensive. Some conventionally grown fruits and vegetables are cleaner than others. You can find the Environmental Working Group's Shopping Guide, which gives you the current Clean 15 and Dirty Dozen—those foods grown with the least and most pesticides—as well as other great shopping tips at www.ewg.org/foodnews/

- Buy locally and seasonally. Does it make sense to buy cherries grown in Chile for $8 a pound in December if you live in North America? Or to buy apples in April that were picked unripe and stored in a warehouse for six months? I bet you've bitten into one of those and yelled at it for tasting so bland and mealy. (Tell me I'm not the only one who does that.) You can save money and get the tastiest produce by buying food that was grown just miles from where you live. Farmers' markets are the best source for the freshest food at the best prices, so scout around and stock up on what's in season in your area. Since certification can be a lengthy process, some vendors may not be organically certified, but there are many who do not spray their crops with chemicals. You can usually speak to the farmers about their farming practices and often find that their products are fairly clean.

- Wash your produce with grapefruit seed extract (GSE). Even if you buy organic, you need to wash everything you purchase to remove the dirt, parasites, fungus, bacteria, and other microbes we don't want to think about. Organic farms do not use filtered water to irrigate, and some farms are located near busy roads where they get exposed to motor exhaust and brake dust. I wash all my produce in the sink with several drops of GSE. I agitate it quite a bit and then allow it to sit for ten minutes before I rinse. GSE is a concentrated liquid that is included in many fruit and veggie washes, which are fine to use as well. Unfortunately, it does not remove pesticides. To remove the pesticides, you can use 1 teaspoon of activated charcoal for a big bowl of water or 1 tablespoon (10 g) for a whole sink. Add produce and allow it to sit for ten to fifteen minutes and then rinse. If you're willing to shell out the money, a water ozonator, like the Ozone Blaster, does the job of GSE and activated charcoal. It attaches to your faucet and creates sanitizing water on demand.

- Get a refrigerator air purifier. These inexpensive little gizmos will remove odors from your refrigerator as well as extend the life of your produce by several days and sometimes even weeks. It's a great way to save money by keeping your produce from spoiling too quickly. I own the Berry Breeze filter, and it's one of the best investments I've made for my kitchen.

KITCHEN TOOLS

Here are the kitchen tools and utensils I like to keep handy:

- ▶ Blender. A high-speed blender with a tamper, like a Vitamix, will give you the best results with the recipes in this book, but a standard blender will do just fine. You may just have to blend a bit longer to get a better consistency for some of the recipes.
- ▶ Food processor. A seven-cup (1.6 L) food processor is the perfect size for the recipes in this book.
- ▶ Juicer. This one is recommended but not required, especially if you already have a high-speed blender. The best juicer is the one that you'll actually use, so look for one that is simple to use and clean. I've had an Omega 8005 for seven years and still love it.
- ▶ Chef's knife and sharpener
- ▶ Large wooden or bamboo cutting board
- ▶ Measuring cups and spoons
- ▶ Nut milk bag for making nut and coconut milks
- ▶ Handy utensils like a spatula, peeler, whisk, hand grater, julienne slicer, citrus reamer, microplane, a handheld mandoline, and a spiralizer for making vegetable noodles

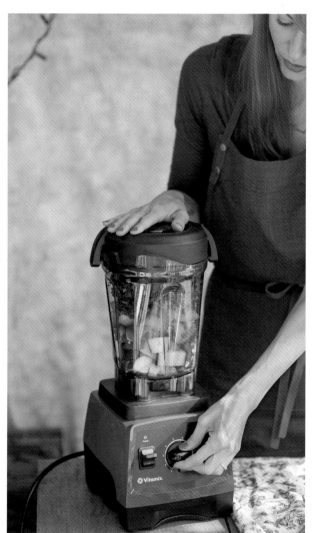

RAW KITCHEN BASICS

There are three things you'll find in almost every raw food kitchen: mason jars, sprouted nuts, and coconuts.

MASON JARS. Get them. Use them. Love them. I'm crazy about my mason jar collection. I have classic and vintage Ball and Kerr jars as well as Italian Bormioli Rocco and German Weck jars of various sizes. I use mason jars not only to drink and store my smoothies, nut milks, and soups, but also for storage of nuts, seeds, and seasonings, and fermenting of kefir, kvass, and cultured vegetables. If you buy bulk items, transfer them to jars instead of storing them in plastic bags. The jars keep food fresh longer, keep the bugs out, and are easier to organize in your pantry.

ACTIVATE SEEDS AND NUTS. Just like the seeds planted in a garden need to be watered to activate life, we need to activate our seeds and nuts before consuming them. By soaking them in water for several hours, we bring them to life and kick up their nutrient content, but most importantly soaking them helps remove the antinutrients like enzyme inhibitors, phytic acid, and tannins that hinder digestibility and block mineral absorption. You'll also notice they taste much better after soaking as the bitterness, especially from nuts like walnuts, is removed. You'll find that almonds actually taste sweet, especially once you remove the skins. Some recipes will call for soaked nuts. See page 71 for instructions and soak times.

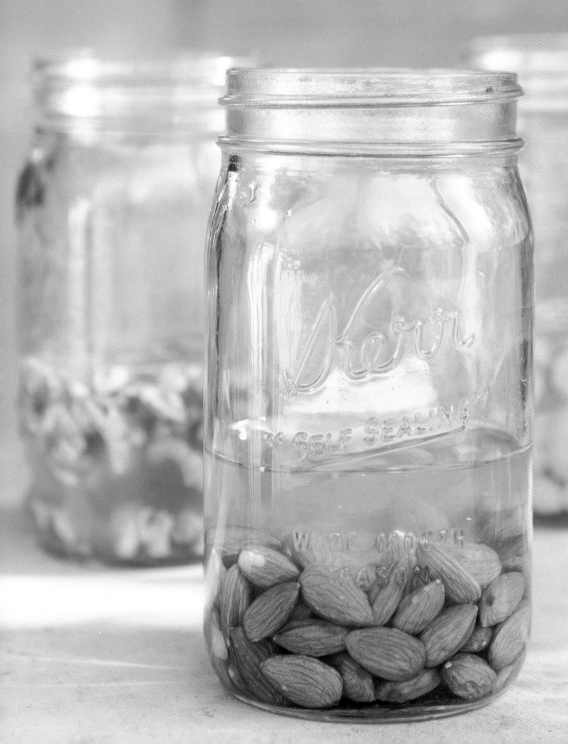

YOUNG THAI COCONUTS. *Coconuts are one of my favorite ingredients to work with. Don't be intimidated by their tough exterior; they are worth the effort. And don't mistake these for the brown fuzzy mature coconuts that have very thick, dry meat and little water. Young Thai coconuts contain soft meat and around 1 to 2 cups (235 to 475 ml) of water. Look for ones with a soft, spongy husk and no dark, purple spots or cracks on the bottom. Here are three ways to crack a coconut:*

METHOD 1: KNIFE AND CLEAVER

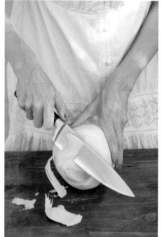 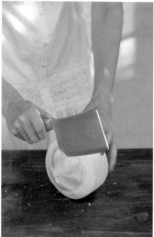 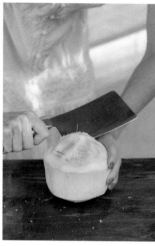 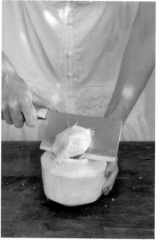

| Use a sharp knife to remove the husk from the top portion or cone of the coconut, exposing the inner hard shell. | Turn the coconut on its side and hold firmly from the bottom. With the heel of a sharp cleaver, aim for the outermost part of the exposed shell and give it a strong whack. It may take a few tries depending on the coconut. | Once you have the cleaver's heel firmly in the shell, turn the coconut back on its base and lift the cleaver to create a flap. This will happen very naturally as the crack will always create a circle. | With a nice grip on the coconut, pry open and pop the top off. |

IMPORTANT

Stay focused when using a cleaver. Do not raise your arm above your head or have your fingers exposed anywhere near the target.

METHOD 2: CLEAVER ONLY

If you have good arm strength, you can give the top of the cone four to five good whacks in a circular fashion. Make sure the coconut is sitting on a firm surface and your free hand is nowhere near it.

METHOD 3: COCO JACK

This is the best contraption I have ever used to open coconuts. It's a two-piece set that includes a mallet and a round metal blade with a handle (the coco jack).

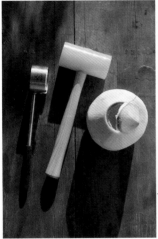 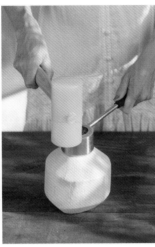 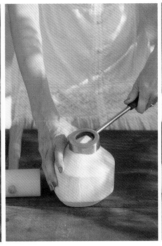 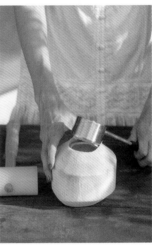

Hold the coco jack firmly in your nondominate hand and the mallet in the other.

Center the coco jack right over the center of the cone. Aim the outside edge of the mallet at the outside edge of the coco jack and give it a few good whacks until it has cut through the shell.

Lift up the handle and insert your finger through the center to dislodge the top of the husk.

ONCE THE COCONUT IS OPEN . . .

1. Pour the coconut water through a fine strainer or sieve to remove any shell pieces.
2. The water should be clear or slightly cloudy and taste sweet. If it is purple, very cloudy, or smells off, you should discard the whole coconut. Always do a taste test before using in a recipe.
3. Store the water in the refrigerator and use within 4 to 5 days or freeze for several weeks in a mason jar.

SCRAPING THE MEAT

1. Use a rubber spatula to scrape out the meat. depending on the coconut, you will have meat ranging from very gelatinous to thick and firm.
2. Remove any bits of shell with a paring knife. Coconut meat will last about 4 to 5 days in the refrigerator or for several weeks in the freezer in a mason jar.

SUPPLEMENTS AND HERBS

Though this book emphasizes food as a means for detoxification, we can also benefit from a little help from Mother Nature's medicine cabinet. The following are natural supplements that can support the detoxification process as you follow this diet. You don't need to take everything on this list, but see if anything resonates positively with you as you read on.

ZEOLITE

Zeolite is a negatively charged, naturally occurring mineral compound that has an affinity for attracting positively charged heavy metals and environmental toxins. It has been shown to neutralize carcinogenic free radicals like the ones created from grilled and charred foods, as well as trapping microbes like bacteria, viruses, and yeasts. Once the zeolite has trapped a toxin in its structure, it is eliminated through the bowels and urine. It's completely safe and nontoxic and has no known side effects. It can be taken daily for everyday detox.

PROBIOTICS

A probiotic first thing in the morning or last thing at night is a great way to help repopulate the gut with healthy flora. Look for ones that contain several different strains of bacteria. I also recommend adding fermented foods like sauerkraut and Beet Kvass (page 69) to your meals to help digest and assimilate your food better. Gut bacteria are essential for breaking down food in the intestines. It's also important to make sure the good guys outnumber the bad guys, like candida. If a probiotic makes you feel bloated and gassy, switch to another brand. Certain strains can aggravate small intestinal bacterial overgrowth (SIBO) if you have it. Most people do very well with Prescript-Assist, which is made from soil-based microorganisms, or SBOs. Take it daily.

MILK THISTLE

The health benefits of milk thistle are largely found in its bioflavonoid complex, silymarin. A powerful antioxidant, it helps protect liver cells by reducing oxidative stress and preventing toxins from entering the liver and also by neutralizing toxins that are already there. It also increases glutathione by more than 35% as well as increases bile production and antioxidant activity, which helps the cleansing function of the liver. Some preliminary studies show milk thistle may also help regenerate damaged liver cells. It's best for short-term use.

CHLORELLA

Chlorella is a single-celled microalgae with a unique molecular structure that bonds with heavy metals, chemicals, and pesticides. Because it is high in chlorophyll, it cleanses and oxygenates the blood. In fact, it has forty times more chlorophyll than wheatgrass juice. It's high pH level makes it great for gut healing as it creates an alkaline environment for good bacteria to thrive in, thereby improving digestion. Purchase chlorella as a powder or in tablet form and make sure it's labeled as broken cell wall chlorella, or else you won't be able to assimilate it. Also, make sure it is grown in an area free of pollution as it can easily absorb toxins from its surrounding area. Chlorella is best taken in the morning with food and can be used safely for everyday detox.

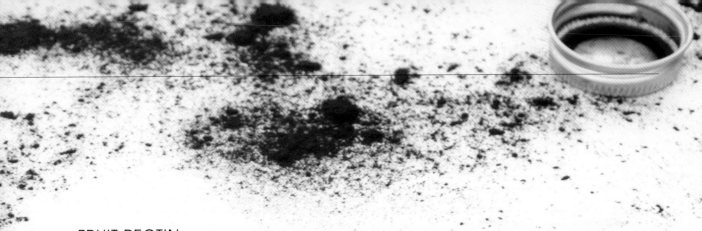

FRUIT PECTIN

Pectin is a soluble fiber found predominately in the skin of fruits and vegetables, especially citrus and apple peels, that is very effective at pulling heavy metals, radioactive isotopes, and other environmental toxins from the gut. Pectin is also a good prebiotic—that is, it feeds beneficial bacteria, which can aid in resolving constipation and diarrhea. Though you'll be eating a lot of pectin on this cleanse, you can also add 5 mg of a pectin supplement per day if you suspect heavy metal toxicity and want a more powerful chelator.

IODINE

Iodine is an essential mineral needed in every cell of our body. Our thyroid is one of many glands and organs that need iodine to help the body function, but it is also the one that is most affected by environmental toxins. When the body is deficient in iodine, cell receptors in the thyroid will absorb heavy metals and halogens, such as bromine, fluorine, and chlorine. Bromine is found in commercial bread, while fluorine, such as sodium fluoride, is found in toothpaste and tap water, and chlorine is found in our water supply, as well. The iodine receptors can also absorb radioactive iodide from leaking nuclear power plants as well as methyl iodide, a very toxic and heavily used pesticide. Iodine supplementation can flush out these toxins as well as chelate heavy metals such as mercury, lead, aluminum, and cadmium. I recommend 400 mcg to 2,000 mcg of nascent iodine per day. This can be used safely for everyday detox and health maintenance.

OIL OF OREGANO

Oil of oregano is a powerful antiviral, antibacterial, antifungal, and antiparasitic compound that is excellent for gut healing. It's very effective at eradicating candida in the large intestines, healing internal and exterior infections, and boosting the immune system. Look for *oreganum vulgare,* or wild oregano, which is the most powerful variety. You can find it encapsulated or as a liquid, but the best is in a whole food supplement form. Beware that liquid extracts are extremely potent and spicy and should be diluted with carrier oil like olive oil or water. Whole food form does not wipe out good bacteria in the gut and is safe for long-term use.

OTHER SUPPLEMENTATION

You do not need to load up on your usual supplements during this detox, but if you regularly take supplements like a multivitamin or green powder, you may continue to do so while detoxing if you so choose, provided that it is a whole food supplement and does not consist of synthetic vitamins. Whole food supplements are becoming more and more the norm, but check the labels. If the label lists folic acid instead of folate, ascorbic acid instead of whole food vitamin C, or cyanobalamin instead of methylcobalamin for B_{12}, you'll know that you are not dealing with a high-quality supplement. These are synthetics that are not bioavailable to the body and will simply be excreted.

DETOX TECHNIQUES

Besides eating cleansing foods and taking herbs and supplements, there are other techniques to get a deeper detox. Incorporate as much as you can from these to get the most out of your raw food cleanse.

EXERCISE

Mild to moderate exercise is a great way to get your lymphatic system going. The main function of the lymphatic system is to move the lymph, a clear fluid containing white blood cells, throughout the body to remove toxins and other unwanted materials. Exercise also pumps blood throughout the body more quickly, encouraging deep cleansing breaths and helping to activate peristalsis. The best exercises to do during a cleanse are walking, rebounding, cycling, elliptical, yoga, and qigong. I don't recommend anything strenuous during your detox since you will be taking in less calories and protein than usual. In general, think of detoxification as a time of rest and relaxation with some bursts of exercise.

DRY SKIN BRUSHING

Dry skin brushing is another way to stimulate the lymphatic system in a gentle, self-caring way. Simply take a coarse, natural-bristle brush and run it softly over your skin, starting at your feet and hands and working toward your heart. It's a light stroking motion, so don't be too abrasive. Just give it a nice, soft scratch in one direction. It will feel unusual at first, but soon you will look forward to it and even desire a coarser brush. Besides stimulating the lymph, you will also be exfoliating dead skin and increasing circulation. Do this for about two to five minutes before you jump into the shower.

SAUNA

Sweating is a great way to move toxins out, particularly when it's done using an infrared sauna. Infrared light penetrates the skin and creates a deep sweat without heating the surrounding air, allowing you to have longer sessions. Start with ten minutes and work your way up to thirty to forty-five minutes, making sure to drink plenty of water. Leave immediately if you feel nauseated or light-headed. Saunas are serious detoxifiers and can make you feel worse if you're very toxic. I prefer to do them at night as they're very relaxing and help me get the best night's sleep ever.

SAUNA DETOX TIPS:

To get the most out of your sauna session, combine it with niacin (vitamin B_3) and rebounding.

Purchase flushing niacin that is not time released. You want the flushing to stimulate the release of toxins from the fat cells (lipolysis). Start with 50 to 100 mg and work your way up slowly. Don't take too much or you will be fantastically hot, itchy, and red as a lobster. Take it about one hour before your sauna session.

While waiting for the niacin to kick in, jump on your rebounder for five to twenty minutes or, if you don't own one, you can jump rope or do jumping jacks. Really, any movement is helpful, but the up and down movement is great for getting the lymphatic system moving.

After rebounding, you can take a dose of zeolites, chlorella, fruit pectin, or activated charcoal to help mop up some of the toxins in the GI tract that will be released.

During your session, use the quiet time to meditate, pray, or listen to soft music or guided meditation. Some people report that they sweat more when meditating. Again, drink plenty of water before, during, and after your sauna session and don't overdo it.

ENEMAS AND COLON HYDROTHERAPY

Enemas can be done at home and are easy and pain-less to administer. It's more of an implant, as you only hold about 1 to 2 cups (235 to 475 ml) water (or more for the advanced people) for about fifteen minutes and then release. You can use purified water, wheatgrass juice, or even coffee, depending on what you want to achieve.

TO ADMINISTER A WATER ENEMA YOU'LL NEED:

- An enema bag or bucket. You can find one at your local pharmacy drugstore or online.
- Coconut oil for lubrication
- An old towel
- Yoga mat (optional)
- 1 to 2 quarts (1 to 2 L) purified water, warmed to body temperature (around 98°F or 37°C)

1. Make sure the hose nozzle is completely closed before you fill it up.
2. Apply a little coconut oil to the end of the insertion tube.
3. While you're on your back, gently insert the tube no more than 3 inches (7.5 cm).
4. Slowly release the hose nozzle and allow the liquid to flow until you feel full but comfortable. The higher the bag, the faster the liquid will flow, so take your time with it and breathe. If you feel a cramp, stop. Breathe and continue when you're ready.
5. Remove the tube and continue lying on your back and massage your abdomen in a clockwise direction to help loosen blockages in the colon.
6. You may only be able to hold it for a few minutes, but eventually work your way up to fifteen minutes before you release.
7. When you're ready, hop on the toilet and release. Repeat a couple more times if desired.

Colonics, on the other hand, need to be done with a professional colon hydrotherapist, but they are much more effective than an enema since they bathe the entire colon. The session usually takes about an hour, but you will have, on average, six bowel movements. Removing this excess waste will give you enormous energy, better digestion, restful sleep, a flatter tummy, and a clearer complexion. I recommend scheduling a session before, during, and after your cleanse. You don't want to be eliminating toxins from the liver only to have them sit in the colon for several days because you're constipated.

ENEMA VARIATIONS:

Water is used if you only want to stimulate peristalsis and unclog the drain, so to speak.

Wheatgrass is used when you want to detoxify and strengthen the colon. The hemorrhoidal vein absorbs the nutrients and brings them into the bloodstream, where it oxygenates the blood. After it passes through the colon, it goes to the liver, where it stimulates de-toxification. You need only about 2 to 6 ounces (60 to 175 ml) of fresh wheatgrass juice straight up or diluted with water, or mix 1 teaspoon of powdered wheatgrass juice into half a quart (0.5 L) of water.

Coffee enemas can also be very powerful, as they help the liver to produce glutathione as well as stimulate bile from the gallbladder and stimulate detoxification. They have been used extensively in Gerson cancer therapy. The Gerson website provides further informa-tion on how to do a coffee enema properly (www. gerson.org/gerpress).

SIMPLE CLEANSING TIP:
Whenever I need to do an enema, I lay down a yoga mat and cover it with a towel on my bathroom floor. I hang the enema bag from a hook on the back of the bathroom door and listen to music or health podcasts to pass the time.

PRE-GAME

Before you jump in head first, there are a few things to get in order:

1. WEAN YOURSELF OFF COFFEE

If you have a coffee/caffeine addiction, it's a good idea to start weaning yourself from it before you start the cleanse. The only coffee allowed on this cleanse is via an enema, so reduce your intake over a couple of weeks to prevent headache withdrawals and acclimate your body to not having stimulants. I do allow a little bit of green matcha tea and raw cacao to get you through the energy slumps if you need to. Stimulants are not a part of the detox, and if you go cold turkey, you're likely to have some excruciating headaches and fatigue. The best way to avoid withdrawal is to slowly reduce your daily intake. If you normally drink three cups of coffee a day, substitute one cup (the last cup of the day) with an herbal tea or coffee substitute such as roasted dandelion root or the nourishing Adrenal Elixir (page 76). After two to three days, substitute another cup with an alternative. A few days later, reduce to drinking half a cup of coffee or just substitute entirely. After a few more days, you should be able to function well without caffeine. If you're still struggling, try the Matcha Boost (page 78).

2. CLEAN OUT THE PANTRY

Throw out any junk food or items not on the cleanse that you feel you cannot live without. This cleanse can be challenging if you have particular food addictions. If there is a food you tend to binge on, get rid of it so it doesn't seduce you when you're feeling weak. Another thing to start weaning yourself off of is junk food. Just like coffee can be physically addicting, so can chemically laced processed foods. These foods are purposely designed to make you want to eat them over and over again. Just like my suggestion for coffee, decrease your intake or find healthy substitutes. Try kale chips and raw sweets instead of potato chips and candy, naturally flavored soda water over cola, and coconut milk ice cream instead of pasteurized, hormone-filled dairy ice cream. These delicious substitutes can be found at most health food stores.

3. BULK IT UP

If your diet lacks fiber, jumping into this 100 percent could be a shock to your digestive tract and lead to uncomfortable bloating. Before you start the cleanse full-on, start introducing more fiber into your diet. You can practice some of the recipes in this book or just start adding salads and smoothies of your choice for a week or two before you begin.

4. GET THINGS MOVING

If your digestive system is sluggish and you are suffering from chronic constipation, you will want to fix this before starting the cleanse. It's essential for you to be able to remove toxins efficiently every day or else you will reintroduce toxins into your body. See the section on digestion for tips on how to relieve constipation (page 15).

5. PLAN

Read through this book, find recipes you like, and get all the items you need to make it happen. Having your weekly menu written down, your shopping list in place, your schedule cleared, and a positive mind-set will ensure your success. With your game plan worked out, you can get focused and excited about the amazing health journey you're about to embark on.

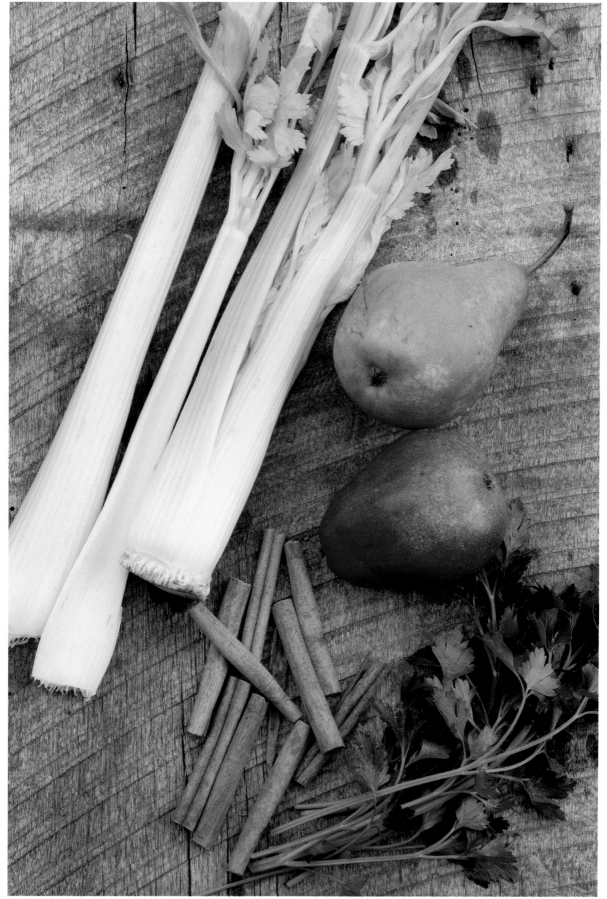

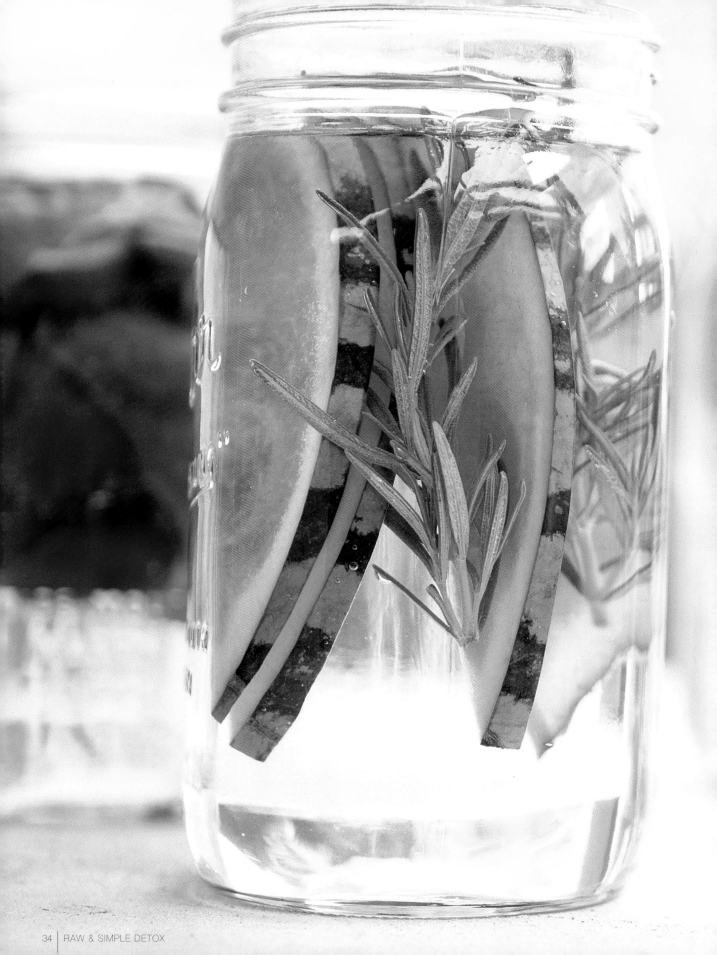

CHAPTER 3
THE RAW & SIMPLE DETOX PLAN

This plan has worked for many of my coaching clients as well as myself, but just as there is no one-size-fits-all diet, there is no one way to cleanse, either. Use my plan as a starting point and template and adjust it to fit your personal needs, goals, and limitations. Some aspects may be too time-consuming or overwhelming for you right now, or certain recommendations may not fit your unique bio-individuality. Some folks might need a deeper or more specific detox. Some have digestive disorders that may not be able to handle raw foods. There is only so much I can fit into one book, so I am sharing what works for many people. Take what resonates and go with it.

GO GREEN!

I hope you like the color green because the majority of your cleansing protocol is going to be gloriously green. Basically, we're going to fill our body with chlorophyll, aka liquid sunshine. Chlorophyll is the pigment in green leaves that absorbs sunlight and converts it to energy. Energy that you will consume in juices, smoothies, soups, and salads. The benefits are many, such as replenishing our red blood cells, carrying oxygen to all our tissues and cells, and neutralizing free radicals. It's also anticarcinogenic and anti-inflammatory and a chelator of heavy metals. Amazingly, the molecular structure is almost identical to hemoglobin except its center atom is magnesium instead of iron. Magnesium is one of the most important minerals our body needs and, yet, most of us are depleted. Greens also contain calcium, potassium, manganese, and folate, which are essential to good health, as well as a fair amount of protein. They also contain omega-3 essential fatty acids, which are also anti-inflammatory, contribute to heart and brain health, and lower the risk of stroke by reducing blood clotting, among many other wonderful health-promoting benefits. So don't fear the green stuff; it's what makes the magic happen. Let's get started!

CLEANSING WITH YOUR CIRCADIAN RHYTHM

All of nature operates on a twenty-four-hour biological clock: The Earth's rotation, daylight and darkness, and ocean tides—but also all living organisms from single-celled to plants to animals to humans. Life ebbs and flows in a biological pattern called circadian (from the Latin *circa*, meaning "about," and *diem*, "day") rhythm. All creatures have optimal times of the day that are best for tissue growth and repair, rest and physical activity, and eating and elimination. By aligning ourselves with these peak times, we can maximize our overall health, strength, hormonal balance, and brain power.

Scientists first started documenting circadian rhythm in the eighteenth century, but traditional Chinese medical texts and ancient Indian Ayurvedic scholars and yogis were already well aware of this phenomenon centuries earlier. They made being in sync with nature an art form—something that is completely lost in our modern society. There is much that we can learn about these ancient healing systems that are still practiced today. Both Western and Eastern health systems offer some insight into how to optimally eat, digest, and rest—all of which I have incorporated into this plan—but it is really all about being in tune with nature's built-in cleansing system.

JUICY MORNINGS

The morning is a time of purification and rehydration. This is the longest period that we have gone without eating or drinking. Our digestion is in a sleepy state, so it's important that we hydrate before we put food in our mouths. Begin the day with a cleansing Lemon Water drink (page 75). Make it fancy or simple, but use hot or room-temperature water for your first drink of the day. Cold water can slow your body's digestive processes, and in this program, we're all about making digestion work as efficiently as possible. This lemony libation stimulates the liver, encourages the production of bile, enhances enzyme function, and, since it's high in vitamin C, boosts the immune system as well as neutralizes pathogens and free radicals. It also hydrates the body and flushes the kidneys, which is crucial when cleansing. Staying hydrated will help curb your appetite, keep your energy up, and induce peristalsis. You can drink this throughout the day as well. Alternatively, you could have herbal tea at this time, one of the warm elixirs like Warm Turmeric Milk (page 80), or just 8 to 16 ounces (235 to 475 ml) of room-temperature water.

Go on with the rest of your morning routine like exercising, meditating, dry brushing, etc. When you begin to feel hunger, juice up with a 16- to 32-ounce (475 to 946 ml) vegetable juice like Everyday Detox (page 55). By removing the fiber, we get pure nutrients into our body without having to digest them. This is very beneficial for those who have impaired digestion or trouble absorbing the nutrients from food. A morning juice replenishes the tissues with minerals and floods your system with chlorophyll to oxygenate your blood. Getting all those rich nutrients early in the day will also help calm some of those naughty food cravings, if you suffer from them.

Twenty minutes after your juice, you can eat something light and easy-to-digest like fruit, chia pudding, a sweet or savory smoothie, or just 1 tablespoon (14 g) of coconut oil. You can stick with an all-juice breakfast for a deeper cleanse or "break the fast" with solids to slow the cleansing. Listen to your body and do what feels best.

For example, your breakfast could be:

FOR A LIGHT CLEANSE:
16 ounces (475 ml) or more of green vegetable juice
Plus a smoothie, Strawberry Chia Parfait (page 130), or fruit with or without Coconut Yogurt (page 168), or a
   few store-bought raw crackers with Power Pesto Spread (page 166) if you need something heartier
Optional: Add an elixir or tonic.

FOR A DEEP CLEANSE:
32 ounces (946 ml) of green vegetable juice
Optional: 1 tablespoon (14 g) of coconut oil
Optional: Add an elixir or tonic like Beet Kvass (page 69) or Turmeric Tonic (page 76).

SIMPLE CLEANSING TIP:
Really try to implement juice first thing in the day, but if it's not possible, have a veggie green smoothie like Simple Savory Smoothie (page 66) for breakfast so you still get plenty of greens and minerals to start your day supercharged.

LUNCH FEAST

Ayurvedic principles teach us that just as the sun's fire peaks in the middle of the day, so does our digestive fire—so make lunch your biggest meal of the day. The body can process big meals better during the day when we are awake and active than at night when we are winding down. Late meals can interfere with detoxification, hormone balance, and fat burning. A recent study published in the *International Journal of Obesity* found that people who eat bigger meals earlier in the day lose more weight.

Make sure to eat until you're satisfied, but don't use that as an excuse to binge. Chew your food slowly and mindfully and when you feel like you're about 80 percent full, stop eating. The recipes in this book are not likely to cause you to go into a food coma, but it's still a good practice to not overdo it. Even though I advocate a raw vegan detox diet, I have worked with clients who simply cannot function without some animal protein. If this is you, then you may add a serving of wild caught fish at this meal if you need. An example of a lunch feast would be:

FOR A LIGHT CLEANSE:
Large salad or wrap
Optional: Add a soup and/or detoxifying treat

FOR A DEEP CLEANSE:
Large smoothie, soup, or 32-ounce (946 ml) juice

BLENDED DINNERS

As daylight begins to fade, our digestive system begins to slow down. This is the ideal time for a light meal like a soup or veggie-based smoothie like Coco Greens (page 63) or Simple Savory Smoothie (page 66). Even when I'm not cleansing, I always recommend blended meals as the last meal of the day. It will fill you up but also not be so heavy as to make you sluggish and tired. In fact, you will probably have a good amount of energy till bedtime and will sleep soundly because your digestive system won't have to work so hard.

FOR A LIGHT CLEANSE:
Soup or vegetable smoothie

FOR A DEEP CLEANSE:
32-ounce (946 ml) vegetable juice

Nighttime is when most of the cleansing takes place. According to the "Chinese clock," our liver is most active between 1 a.m. and 3 a.m. Because we are resting and our digestion is getting a break from our light dinner, the body has more energy to rebuild tissue, recharge the brain, and reset insulin receptors and cortisol and leptin levels. At night we also release the largest amount of human growth hormone, which helps regenerate the liver. All the nutrients, antioxidants, and easy-to-digest meals help maximize our nighttime restoration and natural cleansing process.

From your Blended Dinner up until the Lunch Feast the next day, unless you eat solid foods with your morning juice, you will be in a fasting state. The majority of your detox will be happening while you sleep and in the morning. What could be easier?

FOR THOSE WHO WANT TO FOLLOW A DEEP JUICE CLEANSE:

You may want to include an extra 32-ounce (946 ml) juice (or more) per day to make sure you are getting enough calories. Spread them throughout the day as desired. When you end your cleanse, reintroduce solid food slowly, starting with smoothies and fruit and then move on to salads and cooked vegetables. Eating a big meal right after a juice fast will be very hard on the digestive system. If you do a ten-day juice fast, take five days to get back to eating regularly.

THE DAILY DETOX PLAN

- Lemon Water (page 75) or herbal tea upon rising

- Breakfast: 16 to 32 ounces (475 to 946 ml) vegetable juice; (optional) solid but easy-to-digest food, if needed, such as fruit, chia pudding, or smoothie; (optional) tonic or elixir

- Lunch: main dish, big salad, or blended meal

- Snack (optional): detoxifying treat, fruit, juice, tonic, elixir, crudité with dip, or tea

- Dinner: blended meal, such as a soup or smoothie

- Nighttime (optional): tea, tonic, or elixir

WHEN TO START A RAW DETOX

I live in Southern California, where the weather is warm for most of the year and where the majority of the fruit, vegetables, and nuts in America are grown. So eating seasonally and locally means I get to eat salads and smoothies pretty much all the time. For those who live where there are actually four seasons, I recommend doing a raw detox in the spring, summer, or fall. Spring and fall are the seasons of change and are regarded as optimum times for detoxification, according to Ayurveda. If you choose to do it in the summer, hot weather will make you crave cooling foods and the availability of ingredients will be plentiful and less expensive. Summer has always been my favorite time to cleanse for this reason. Of course, you can still detox during the cooler months, but an all-raw diet would not be ideal. See my section on how to follow a winter detox on page 52.

Besides the seasonal factor, the best time to kick off your cleanse is over a weekend when you don't have a lot of pressing demands. Give yourself space to do this right. Clear your schedule, get a babysitter, and get into a zone where you can completely focus on yourself, at least for a couple of days. The beginning is the most challenging, but once you get the hang of making new recipes, eating new foods, and experiencing new sensations, you'll get into a flow. Soon you'll be able to make recipes in a flash, your energy will be soaring, and you will have no problem incorporating the cleanse into your daily routine.

HOW LONG SHOULD I DETOX?

Since this is not as deep of a cleanse as juice fasting, you could follow this detox safely for a few days or a few weeks. That said, I recommend fourteen to twenty-one days—this is a long enough time to create some lasting health benefits. But use good judgment on how long you should detox. If you're really toxic, you may want to detox for three weeks but follow a lighter cleanse by eating more solid foods. If you've cleansed before or already eat a clean diet, then follow it for a week, but follow the deep cleanse plan with more juices and less solid foods. Even a day or two can help reset your system after a binge or holiday blowout. Stick to it as long as you see and feel your health improving.

WHAT CAN I EXPECT?

Depending on your toxicity and how well your body responds to a raw food diet, your experience could be very similar to what I describe here or very different. Not everyone has the same results, but prepare yourself for the following sensations.

THE FIRST THREE DAYS

Expect intense food cravings and possible headaches from withdrawal from caffeine, sugar, and processed foods if you did not give yourself enough time to kick the habit. Mood shifts are common when adjusting to a new diet. It's only temporary. Energy levels will ebb and flow at this time, too, as you get accustomed. You may also have gas and bloating from all the added fiber, but this could indicate a sluggish constitution, an intolerance to fructose, or dysbiosis as well.

DAYS 4 to 7

You should start to feel greatly energized, but you could also be noticing skin rashes and breakouts as your body is starting to move toxins out via the skin. This could come and go during the whole cleanse. Also, expect to feel more emotional. Traditional Chinese medicine states that anger is stored in the liver. As your liver becomes less burdened, pent-up emotions will begin to release. A good cry could creep up on you when you least expect it. Let it out if you're alone and allow emotional healing to take place.

DAYS 8 to 10

You should start to notice significant changes in sugar cravings if you have been following a low-glycemic plan. Your tummy should be flatter and you should be feeling radiant the majority of the time. The cleanse should feel comfortable at this time and digestion should be regular, with two to three movements a day.

DAY 11 AND BEYOND

Cravings will still rear their heads now and then, but this is the point where you should be coasting along.

THE HERZHEIMER REACTION

A healing crisis, also known as the Herzheimer reaction, happens when the cells and liver release waste faster than the body can eliminate it. It can also happen as pathogenic organisms, such as candida, begin to die off. For most people, symptoms will be mild, but can include fatigue, headaches, nausea, loose stools, joint pain, skin rashes, hot flashes, or the chills. It's normal to go from feeling great to not so great, but you should stop the cleanse immediately if you feel chronically ill or have vomiting, intestinal pain, or diarrhea.

HOW MUCH SHOULD YOU EAT?

You do not need to count calories or obsess about portion size. The majority of the recipes are low-calorie, so even if you ate two to three servings you would be well within your dietary calorie range. The only meal that is hearty will be the Lunch Feast, while breakfast and dinner should be lighter. Even the light meals should be satisfying, but never to the point of feeling stuffed. Remember: Eat until you are 80 percent full and then stop.

DON'T FEAR THE FAT

Forget the diet myth that fat makes you fat. Actually, good fats are the body's preferred form of energy. They satiate your appetite, lubricate your skin, and help you to absorb fat-soluble vitamins like A, D, E, and K. Fats are essential for a detox diet because they promote the release of bile from the bladder, allowing for the elimination of toxins from the body. Good fats are the ones used in this book, like coconut, avocado, nuts, seeds, and olive oil. They also happen to be super delicious. And the really great news is most people can thrive on a higher fat diet and lose weight in the process, particularly if carbohydrates are kept low. I'm not advocating a ketogenic diet where you eat mainly fat and a low amount of protein and carbohydrates to enter a ketogenic fat-burning state. We still want to keep the fat intake in moderation while cleansing so that the liver can spend most of its energy on detoxification.

That being said, there are some who don't do as well with fats. Those with gallstones or removed gallbladders, irritable bowel syndrome, pancreatitis, liver disease, or any other liver impairment will want to go with the low- to no-fat recipes in this book or just reduce or omit the fats from the recipes as needed.

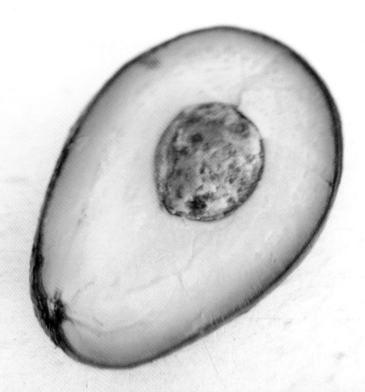

PROTEIN NEEDS

A raw diet, especially one that includes blended greens, can provide a sufficient amount of protein for most people. All the vegetables, seeds, and nuts you'll be enjoying contain some amount of protein. Even fruit contains trace amounts of protein. You can also get protein from superfoods like spirulina and bee pollen, which are composed of about 60 percent and 40 percent protein, respectively. Here are a few stats:

Hemp Seeds	3 tablespoons (23 g) = 10 grams
Chia Seeds	3 tablespoons (39 g) = 9 grams
Raw Almonds	1 ounce (28 g) = 6 grams
Sunflower Seeds	1 ounce (28 g) = 6 grams
Fresh Peas	1 cup (150 g) = 6 grams
Raw Tahini	2 tablespoons (30 g) = 5 grams
Cacao Nibs	1 ounce (28 g) = 4 grams
Broccoli	1 cup raw (71 g) = 3 grams
Avocado	1 medium = 3 grams
Goji Berries	1 ounce (28 g) = 3 grams
Kale	1 cup (67 g) = 2 grams

If you're a "protein type" and feel like you're not getting enough on the cleanse, then try adding a vegan protein powder like sprouted brown rice, pea, or hemp protein. You can add these to your smoothies or just blend with Coconut Milk (page 72) or Almond Milk (page 70) for a boost as needed.

If you prefer animal protein, then wild-caught fish is allowed and, ideally, eaten during your Lunch Feast. Best choices are baked or poached salmon, trout, halibut, mackerel, or canned sardines (look for sustainably caught and BPA-free cans). I even included an easy and delicious Almond-Crusted Salmon Filet (page 148) recipe.

GET TO KNOW (AND LOVE) THE DETOX TOP 12

Almost every ingredient I use in this book was specially chosen for its unique health benefits. There are many recurring foods in these recipes that you may appreciate more if you know how powerful they are. Here are a few you'll be seeing a lot of and why I love them:

1. COCONUTS
This is my favorite ingredient in the book. We'll be whipping up lots of tasty recipes using coconut oil, coconut meat, and occasionally the coconut water. Though coconuts do not actually detoxify, they are very supportive for this cleanse and contain many health benefits, the majority of them from the fat content. The medium chain triglycerides, or MCTs, are one of the most excellent and health-promoting fats for human health.

IMMUNE SUPPORT
The fatty acids that comprise coconut oil have antiviral, antibacterial, and antifungal properties. One of these fatty acids, lauric acid, is converted into monolauren, which is the most effective at breaking down the protective lipid coating of pathogens, thereby preventing them from reproducing and proliferating. Coconut oil has been helpful in the treatment of herpes, influenza, measles, and giardia.

IMPROVED GUT HEALTH
This unique ability of monolauren to destroy bacteria makes it very effective at breaking down biofilm in the gut that is produced when colonies of bad bacteria take up shop in the nooks and crannies of your intestines. This is very helpful for those suffering from candida overgrowth and for those who have inflammation caused by microorganisms. Since coconut oil is metabolized easily by the body, it can be very beneficial for people who are not able to digest other fats.

BOOSTS BRAINPOWER
A recent study showed that the medium chain tryglicerides (MCTs) in coconut oil boosts brain function in people with Alzheimer's disease. Our brains primarily use glucose for fuel, but when glucose uptake is impaired (e.g., insulin resistance—think of Alzheimer's as diabetes of the brain), it can utilize the ketone bodies that are created by the liver when coconut oil is consumed instead. Try a tablespoon of coconut oil (14 g) or pure MCT oil whenever you have brain fog. That's pretty much how I wrote this book!

AIDS DIGESTION
Coconut oil helps satiate appetite as well as increase fat burning. It does not spike insulin and is used in the body as a quick source of energy instead of being stored as fat. One study on women with abdominal fat showed noticeable waist-size reduction by adding only 2 tablespoons (28 g) of oil a day to their diet and nothing else. Enjoy a tablespoon (14 g) in the morning with your juice, added to a smoothie or soup, or as a snack.

MOISTURIZES
Go ahead and slather it on your skin as a moisturizer, shaving cream, and makeup remover as well!

(continued on page 44)

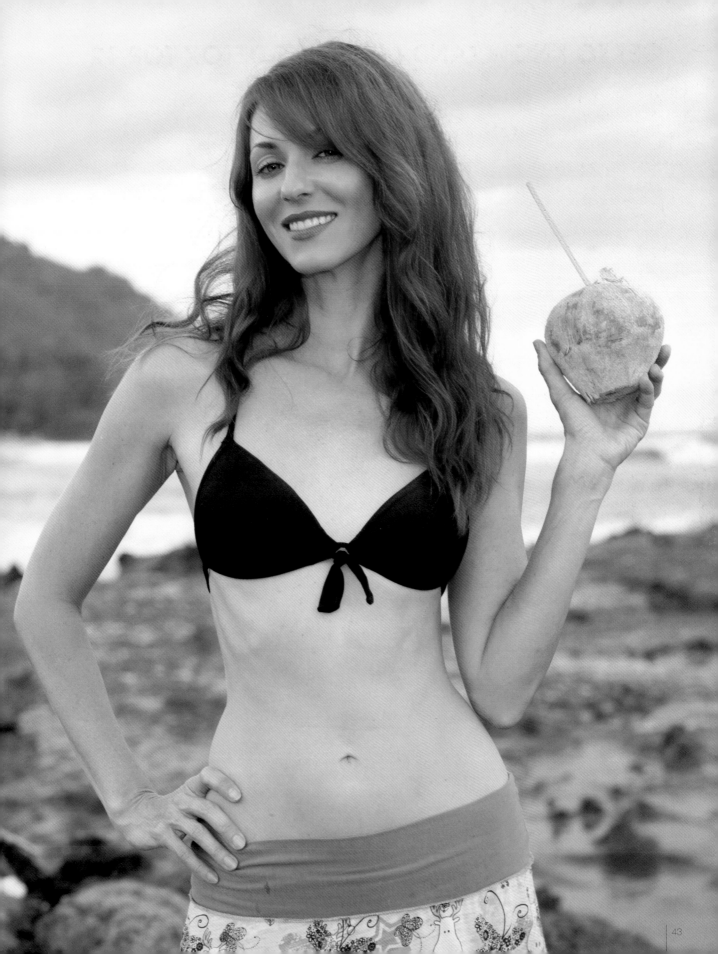

GET TO KNOW (AND LOVE) THE DETOX TOP 12

(continued from page 42)

2. CUCUMBERS What's not to love? They're hydrating, cooling, and delicious. The skin, seeds, and flesh are all high in nutrients, so don't peel and seed them (or just throw the peel and seeds into the juicer!). Cucumbers aid detoxification by helping the kidneys excrete waste and help to reduce inflammation by expelling uric acid from the body. They are very beneficial for those suffering from arthritis, asthma, and gout, and they even help dissolve kidney stones. Cukes are high in silica, which helps strengthen bones, joints, and connective tissues, and is great for skin, nails, hair, and even for slowing hair loss.

3. AVOCADOS Creamy, luscious avocados not only make this cleanse bearable, but they are also fiber- and nutrient-rich powerhouses. They have lots of monounsaturated oleic acid that helps reduce LDL (bad) cholesterol and boost heart health and also contain a good dose of folate, vitamin E, omega-3s, and antioxidants, making them one of the top brain-healthy foods. They're also a good source of glutathione, the master antioxidant that helps support the liver and nervous system and slow aging, and they aid digestion by reducing inflammation in the stomach and small intestine.

4. CILANTRO This culinary herb has one main job and that is as a heavy metal chelator. *Chelate* comes from the Latin word for "claw," so imagine that claw drawing out impurities from your body as you take down your daily juice. Heavy metal toxicity can cause an array of health problems such as brain fog, fatigue, depression, headaches, and other neurological issues, so don't underestimate cilantro's superpower.

SIMPLE CLEANSING TIP: *Cilantro can be so detoxifying that, whenever I have a lot of it, I also take chlorella or pectin to mop up the heavy metals that enter the colon.*

5. APPLES Pectin, the soluble fiber in apples, soaks up heavy metals and other toxins and sweeps them through the intestines. Apples also contain glucaric acid, which helps the body get rid of carcinogens, steroids, and toxins in the liver. Apples are also high in vitamin C, B vitamins, and an array of phytonutrients that are helpful for reducing risk of stroke, breast cancer, diabetes, dementia, and heart disease. Researchers from the University of Oxford in the United Kingdom found that eating an apple every day could be just as effective as statins in preventing vascular deaths among people over fifty.

6. CHIA SEEDS The word chia is Nahuatl for "strength." The ancient Aztec warriors took these cute little seeds with them into battle for energy and endurance. They contain a whopping 3 grams of complete protein and 5 grams of fiber per tablespoon (13 g). The fiber is great for our digestion, but when soaked, chia seeds become very hydrating for the colon and excellent for relieving constipation. The hydrophilic colloidal (liquid-attracting) property of soaked chia seeds makes them easily digestible, even for those with diverticulitis. In fact, hydrophilic colloids have been used in the healing of many digestive problems from sour stomach to intestinal discomfort. It is even beneficial if eaten alongside other foods as a digestive aid. Add chia gel (page 87) to smoothies and other recipes if you have any gastrointestinal issues.

7. LEMONS Mother Nature's all-purpose cleanser helps detoxify the liver, increase the production of bile, cleanse the urinary tract, and improve digestive function. Lemons help destroy pathogenic bacteria, boost the immune system, and are fantastic for repairing skin.

8. GINGER A powerful anti-inflammatory and digestive aid, ginger improves the absorption and assimilation of nutrients and can help heal leaky gut syndrome. Studies show that ginger can reduce inflammation in the colon, lower high blood pressure, and reduce menstrual cramps and may help prevent acetaminophen-induced liver damage. Ginger has been used for over two thousand years as a natural treatment for colds, flu, and nausea. Its antibiotic properties have shown to be even more effective at treating staph infections than antibiotics and can even help prevent intestinal ulcers and inhibit *H. pylori* bacteria in the stomach, which can also cause ulcers. Ginger amplifies turmeric's power, which is why I often use them together in recipes.

9. TURMERIC Curcumin is the powerful anti-inflammatory and antioxidant compound in this bright orange root that is widely used in Ayurveda as a healing food. Studies have shown that it is effective in treating arthritis and depression and reducing the risk of heart disease, cancer, and Alzheimer's disease. It's been used as an effective treatment for inflammatory bowel diseases like Crohn's and ulcerative colitis and helps stimulate bile in the gallbladder, which makes it a great addition to a liver and digestive cleanse.

10. BEETS This vegetable is rich in betalains, phytonutrients that are important for phase two of the liver detoxification process, which are powerful anti-inflammatories and antioxidants. Beets are also high in vitamin K, beta carotene, and folate, have been used as an aphrodisiac and a brain and stamina booster, and have shown to be helpful in lowering blood pressure and counteracting cancerous cell growth.

11. CRUCIFEROUS VEGETABLES I can't list just one member of the Brassica family when they're really a package deal. Broccoli, cauliflower, brussels sprouts, kale, cabbage, radish, bok choy, collard greens, turnips, mustard greens, arugula, and watercress deserve to be called super-veggies because of their anticancer and bad-estrogen-lowering compounds called glucosinolates. Besides their ability to slow the growth of cancer cells, they can also detoxify carcinogens before they damage cells. The sulfur compounds in cruciferous vegetables enhance the liver's detoxification pathways while helping the liver break down and eliminate fat through the bile ducts.

12. GARLIC Used traditionally for its antibacterial, antifungal, and antiviral properties, this healing herb is a powerful anti-inflammatory and antioxidant as well. With more than 150 different health uses, garlic's therapeutic effect comes from its sulfur-containing compounds, such as allicin. As a detox herb, in a recent study, garlic has been shown to chelate lead and boost the body's ability to detox by increasing production of glutathione.

DETOX TRICKS AND TIPS

Here are a few things to help make your health journey the best ever:

1. Keep a journal. Before you begin, write down your health goals and the benefits you will receive when you reach your goal. When I began my first raw food cleanse, I wrote down that I wanted clearer skin. The benefits of clearer skin, for me, would be feeling more beautiful, having confidence when I auditioned in front of the camera, and booking more modeling gigs. Booking more gigs would mean more money and more freedom to do things I love to do. Whenever I needed motivation, I would read over my goals to remind myself why I was doing it. In the end, it paid off exactly like I had hoped. Think about what you want. More energy to start new projects, play with your kids, or get into an exercise routine? Mental clarity to excel at work and get that promotion or write a book or start a blog? It's also great to journal what you eat and record how that food made you feel. You could have underlying food sensitivities you were unaware of until you began getting in tune with your body. Journal your feelings, as well. What emotions are you releasing? What are you grateful for? Do this daily and see how you transform over the course of this cleanse.

2. Don't binge the night before you start your cleanse. This is a popular strategy that will only make your first day tougher. Trust me, I know from experience. Eating a big blowout meal that probably includes every one of the foods you should be avoiding will trigger more food cravings throughout the first few days. If you need a blowout, do it the week before and then make sure you prep by decreasing junk foods and increasing fiber intake.

3. Drink enough fluids. Raw foods are hydrating on their own, but it's still good to flush the kidneys regularly throughout the cleanse with lots of fluids. Staying hydrated with also help curb hunger and cravings. Also, you don't have to only drink water. There are a dozen different beverages you can enjoy in this book besides plain old water.

4. Chill then chew. Always eat when you're in a restful state of mind. If you're upset or stressed, this can impair digestion. Remember that gut-brain connection I mentioned in Chapter 1? What we think affects the nervous system of our gut. If your stomach has ever been "in knots," then you know exactly what I'm talking about. Take ten deep breaths before you dig in to switch your brain from the sympathetic (fight or flight state) to the parasympathetic (rest and recovery state) nervous system. I like to close my eyes and give thanks for the food as well, but I'm a hippy like that. Once you're chilled out, chew that food well. Your stomach doesn't have teeth, so make it easy on your gut by chewing until food becomes liquid. Eat slowly and mindfully, enjoying the flavors, textures, and beauty of living foods.

5. Try not to graze. When we constantly eat, we don't give our digestion enough time to do the work it needs to do. That's why several small meals a day usually won't help dieters lose weight because they are always burning the calories they just ate instead of burning fat. Snacks are allowed, but, ideally, if you can get by without, you would be giving your body a break from the constant work of digesting and thus getting a little deeper of a cleanse, burning more fat, and getting a nice energy boost.

6. You're in control of how deep or light you want to cleanse. If you feel like going deep, stick to juices, soups, and smoothies; if you want to take it slow, eat more solid food. It's perfectly fine to switch gears from day to day or meal to meal. You don't need to suffer. Just listen to your body and go with the flow. You will probably find that on days that are stressful or demanding, you will want more solid food, while on quiet, restful days, you will feel just fine with liquids.

7. Get more sleep. Hit the hay no later than 10 p.m. and try to get at least seven hours of uninterrupted sleep, but eight to nine hours would be ideal. Make sure to block out any extra light coming through your bedroom window and unplug all electronics in your room. Electromagnetic fields (EMF) from household appliances and cell phones can affect your nervous system and interfere with the body's natural healing process. Turn your cell phone off or switch it to airplane mode and don't leave it near your head. If you have a Wi-Fi router in your home, turn it off at night. Sleep is a crucial part of detoxification, hormone balance, brain function, and tissue rejuvenation.

8. Get grounded. You know those EMFs I just told you about? When you're touching the Earth barefoot, you become shielded from them by the negative electron charge of the planet. When we're connected to Earth in this way, all the positive (damaging) ions that have built up or are assaulting us are discharged into the ground. Free radicals are neutralized, inflammation is reduced, blood flow improves, stress and anxiety is lifted, and we can feel a sense of calm and mental clarity. Try to do this for half an hour a day—and get some sunshine while you're at it. We need vitamin D for strong bones, fertility, a good immune system, and disease prevention.

9. Exercise. Earlier I mentioned exercise to keep the blood pumping and the lymph moving, but it also helps improve brain function. I often find I come up with the best ideas when I'm working out. This is because exercise increases blood flow into micro blood vessels in the brain, which are associated with creating new brain cells. Exercise also releases endorphins, which increases mental alertness and cognitive function and creates a sense of well-being, much like coffee does! Don't do anything strenuous, but do a little activity every day.

10. Deal with cravings. Unfortunately, cravings are going to rear their naughty heads over the course of your cleanse. But that's why I gave you detox friendly treats and Italian food recipes! The first thing you need to do when a craving arises is make sure you're getting enough liquids. Dehydration can make you feel hungry, so get that out of the way first. Next, try to change your focus. If you're bored, it's easy to start wanting to snack. Stay busy doing things you're passionate about

and you'll probably forget your cravings. Fatigue can also make you reach for snacks, so make sure you get enough sleep and sneak in some naps if you can, as well. If you feel blood sugar instability is making you snacky, take 100 to 200 mcg of GTF (glucose tolerance factor) chromium three times a day. This has helped curb my sweet tooth big time. If you still need to satisfy some intense food cravings, try this:

• For salty crunch, try some raw crackers or raw kale chips.

• For soda pop, try sparkling mineral water with a couple drops of vanilla stevia for a cream soda or just a squeeze of fresh fruit juice for flavor.

• I've included raw chocolate bark (page 158) and a few different frozen treats as well. If chocolate doesn't help, I don't know what will!

11. Get back on after giving in. So your office decided to have donut week right when you started your cleanse, or you had to attend your friend's big fat Greek wedding, and at your darkest hour you fell off the wagon. No worries. Just get right back on. One meal doesn't mean the cleanse is over or the rest of the day is a free-for-all. Dust yourself off and get back in the game. Let your next meal be damage control and move on.

LOW SUGAR SEVEN-DAY
DETOX MEAL PLAN

This plan is for those who have blood sugar issues or suspect candida overgrowth.

DAY 1

▶ **BREAKFAST:**
Everyday Detox (page 56) (use green apples or stevia); (optional) Simple Savory Smoothie (page 66) or 1 to 2 tablespoons (14 to 28 g) coconut oil

▶ **LUNCH:**
Green Submarine Wrap (page 138)

▶ **Snack (Optional):** Almond Butter Chocolate Bark (page 158)

▶ **DINNER:**
Sopa Verde (page 94)

DAY 2

▶ **BREAKFAST:**
Spicy Garden (page 56); (optional) Strawberry Chia Parfait (page 130) or 1 to 2 tablespoons (14 to 28 g) coconut oil

▶ **LUNCH:**
Greek Salad (page 118)

▶

▶ **DINNER:**
Dinner: Coco Greens (page 63)

DAY 3

▶ **BREAKFAST:**
Heavy Metal Detox (page 57) (use green apples or stevia); (optional) Berry Muesli Cereal (page 132) or 1 to 2 tablespoons (14 to 28 g) coconut oil

▶ **LUNCH:**
Ginger-Miso Veggie Rolls (page 136)

▶ **Snack (Optional):** Coconut-Basil Sorbet (page 156)

▶ **DINNER:**
Cream of Tomato Soup (page 95)

DAY 4

▶ **BREAKFAST:**
▶ Liver Flush (page 57) (use green apples or stevia); (optional) Coco Greens (page 63)
or 1 to 2 tablespoons (14 to 28 g) coconut oil

▶ **LUNCH:**
Zucchini Noodles Al Dente (page 140) with Pesto Sauce (page 166)

▶ **Snack (Optional):** Strawberry Chia Parfait (page 130) with or without fruit

▶ **DINNER:**
Simple Savory Smoothie (page 66)

DAY 5

▶ **BREAKFAST:**
Blood Cleanser (page 57) (use green apples or stevia); (optional) Herby Vegetable Smoothie (page 67)
or 1 to 2 tablespoons (14 to 28 g) coconut oil

▶ **LUNCH:**
The Quickie Salad (page 122)

▶ **Snack (Optional):** Queen of Green Dip (page 169) with crudités

▶ **DINNER:**
Cucumber-Mint Soup (page 91)

DAY 6

▶ **BREAKFAST:**
Everyday Detox (page 56) (use green apples or stevia); (optional) Grapefruit-Avocado Salad (page 122)
or 1 to 2 tablespoons (14 to 28 g) coconut oil

▶ **LUNCH:**
Rustic Raw Lasagna (page 129)

▶ **Snack (Optional):** Strawberry Chia Parfait (page 130)

▶ **DINNER:**
Herby Vegetable Smoothie (page 67)

DAY 7

▶ **BREAKFAST:**
Heavy Metal Detox (page 57) (use green apples or stevia); (optional) Adrenal
Elixir (page 76) or 1 to 2 tablespoons (14 to 28 g) coconut oil

▶ **LUNCH:**
Romaine Fresco Tacos (page 134)

▶ **Snack (Optional):** Botija olives and ¼ cup (36 g) soaked almonds

▶ **DINNER:**
Coconut-Broccoli Shorba (page 96)

LOW FAT SEVEN-DAY
DETOX MEAL PLAN

This is for those who want to follow a low-fat plan. Keep in mind that you may need to eat bigger portions to get enough calories.

DAY 1

▶ **BREAKFAST:**
Coco Greens (page 63); (optional) Strawberry Chia Parfait (page 134)

▶ **LUNCH:**
Zucchini Noodles Al Dente (page 140) with Tomato Marinara (page 167)

▶ **Snack (Optional):** Tropical Bliss Pudding (page 154) (omit tahini if desired) or fruit

▶ **DINNER:**
Sweet Pea, Mint, and Fennel Soup (page 92)

DAY 2

▶ **BREAKFAST:**
Kidney Cleanser (page 56); (optional) We Got the Beet Smoothie (page 59)

▶ **LUNCH:**
Carrot Coleslaw (page 116)

▶ **Snack (Optional):** Fruit

▶ **DINNER:**
Sopa Verde (page 94) without avocado

DAY 3

▶ **BREAKFAST:**
Everyday Detox (page 56); (optional) Papa-Pina Digestive (page 60)

▶ **LUNCH:**
Tabbouleh Salad Wraps (page 142)

▶ **Snack (Optional):** Banana Soft Serve with Raspberry Sauce (page 151)

▶ **DINNER:**
The California Smoothie (page 66)

DAY 4

▶ **BREAKFAST:**
Skin Glow (page 56); (optional) Celery-Pear Pick-Me-Up (page 67)

▶ **LUNCH:**
Middle Eastern Beet Salad (page 116)

▶ **Snack (Optional):** Fiesta Fruit Cup (page 162)

▶ **DINNER:**
Simple Savory Smoothie (page 66)

DAY 5

▶ **BREAKFAST:**
Liver Flush (page 57); (optional) Ginger Spiced Apple Smoothie (page 60)

▶ **LUNCH:**
Green Submarine Wrap (page 138) without avocado

▶ **Snack (Optional):** Fruit

▶ **DINNER:**
Dilly Beet Soup (page 98) (omit or use less avocado)

DAY 6

▶ **BREAKFAST:**
Spicy Garden (page 56); (optional) The California Smoothie (page 66)

▶ **LUNCH:**
Arugula Salad with Jicama, Blood Orange, and Raspberry Vinaigrette (page 105)

▶ **Snack (Optional):** Graperfruit-Ginger Chia Drink (page 86)

▶ **DINNER:**
Curried Seaweed Soup (page 100)

DAY 7

▶ **BREAKFAST:**
Root Juice (page 56); (optional) Raspberry Kombucha Margarita (page 84)

▶ **LUNCH:**
Dandelion-Fennel Salad (page 110)

▶ **Snack (Optional):** Fruit

▶ **DINNER:**
Vegetable Soup (page 103)

WINTER CLEANSE

In the colder months, our body craves warming foods. Fruit smoothies and icy treats are not ideal for our constitution at this time, but warm soups and teas are great, along with gently warmed dishes. I have included a few cooked recipes and several recipes that can be gently warmed in a dehydrator or over the stovetop. For salads and vegetable smoothies, use room-temperature vegetables (just leave them out on the counter for an hour before you prep). You may also add in steamed vegetables seasoned with salt, pepper, and olive oil, or drizzled with one of the dressings from page 126. Here are a list of recipes in the book that would be appropriate for a winter detox.

- Any of the vegetable juices (pages 56 to 57) (room temperature)
- Coconut or nut milk (page 72 or 70)
- Adrenal Elixir (page 76)
- Turmeric Tonic (page 76)
- Warm Turmeric Milk (page 80)
- Matcha Boost (page 78)
- Cold Buster (page 86)
- Lemon Water (page 75) (hot or room temperature)
- Simple Savory Smoothie (page 66) (room temperature)
- Herby Vegetable Smoothie (page 67) (room temperature)
- Sopa Verde (page 94) (room temperature)
- Coconut-Broccoli Shorba (page 96) (gently warmed)
- Dilly Beet Soup (page 98) (gently warmed)
- Cream of Tomato Soup (page 95) (gently warmed)
- Sweet Pea, Mint, and Fennel Soup (page 92) (gently warmed)
- Vegetable Soup (page 103) (cooked)
- Curried Seaweed Soup (page 100) (cooked)

- Shaved Brussels Sprout–Apple Salad with Hazelnuts (page 108) (room temperature)
- Greek Salad (page 118) (room temperature)
- The Quickie Salad (page 122) (room temperature)
- Kale Is Kind Salad (page 114) (room temperature)
- Carrot Coleslaw (page 116) (room temperature)
- Middle Eastern Beet Salad (page 116) (room temperature)
- Chinese Cabbage Salad with Orange Tahini Dressing (page 112) (room temperature)
- Carrot Ribbon Salad (page 106) (room temperature)
- Asian Bok Choy Salad (page 120) (room temperature)
- Zucchini Noodles Al Dente (page 140) (gently warmed)
- Rustic Raw Lasagna (page 129) (room temperature)
- Asian Root Wraps (page 146) (room temperature)
- Sweet and Spicy Kelp Noodles (page 144) (gently warmed)
- Almond-Crusted Salmon Filet (page 148) (cooked)
- Tabbouleh Salad Wrap (page 142) (room temperature)
- Almond Butter Chocolate Bark (page 158)

FOOD SENSITIVITY

Before your cleanse, you may not have noticed food sensitivities. If you've done at least a fourteen-day cleanse and want to reintroduce foods you've been avoiding, you can add one food at a time and note any reactions. Issues could happen as soon as you eat the food or up to seven days later and could include nausea, stomachache, brain fog, skin rash, or headache. Since you're more in tune with your body, you will know what foods to avoid in the future. Keep track in your journal and note if you have any reactions to the foods you used to eat.

MORE RAW AND SIMPLE TIPS

Feeling overwhelmed? I remember that feeling eight years ago when I dove into the raw food diet 100 percent. The biggest issue for most people is finding the time to prepare. Believe me, once you start making these recipes, you will be making them in your sleep. What may take half an hour the first time will take ten or fifteen minutes the next. Here are a few little tricks to help you out:

- Keep it simple. Stick to fast and easy recipes like the Quickie Salad (page 122) or the Simple Savory Smoothie (page 66) when you're busy. In fact, you don't even have to make recipes from my book. You could enjoy a bowl of fruit or a simple garden salad, cucumber slices with a dash of salt and pepper, or some sliced apples with a dollop of nut butter. I'm just giving you inspiration for things to eat so you're not bored. Don't feel like you have to be a gourmet chef every meal of the day. Keeping it simple is a great way to stick to the plan and not burn out.

- Juices are best freshly made, but if you're short on time in the mornings, you can prepare your juice the night before. Store it in a mason jar filled to the very top in the refrigerator. The less oxygen in the jar, the less degradation there will be.

- If preparing the Lunch Feast is too difficult with your work schedule, find a local restaurant that serves big, juicy salads (one that uses organic or local greens, if possible). Bring your own homemade salad dressing or request a house vinaigrette or just olive oil and lemon wedges.

- Though I designed this plan around optimum digestive circadian rhythm, you may find that a Lunch Feast doesn't fit into your work schedule. You can absolutely move your feast to dinner and have a blended lunch instead. This is ideal for people who work busy day jobs and those who find they aren't as hungry during the day.

- You don't have to make it all yourself. Prepackaged produce is not my first choice, but if it helps you stick with the plan, then do it. Buy prepackaged salad greens, prepared salads (toss the dressing if it has any oil besides olive), prepared raw meals, cut-up fruit, and crudités. Give yourself a break and support your local raw food restaurant and juice bar.

LIFE AFTER DETOX

I've equipped you with dozens of healthy lifestyle tips. You may not be able to follow everything in this book, but try to add a couple healthy habits every week. Health is a lifelong journey, so make it a priority. My hope, after you have completed this detox, is that you feel so amazing that you will want to continue to upgrade your health and every area of your life. Whatever dietary path you choose, try to eat as close to nature as possible. Choose real, organic, unprocessed, seasonal, and pastured food. Going back to your old diet will not serve you and will only return you to the place you started.

Stay in sync with nature and live as naturally as possible and know that you can always come back and reboot as needed. If you want more inspiration, easy raw food recipes, and healthy lifestyle tips, check out my books *Going Raw* and *Raw & Simple*.

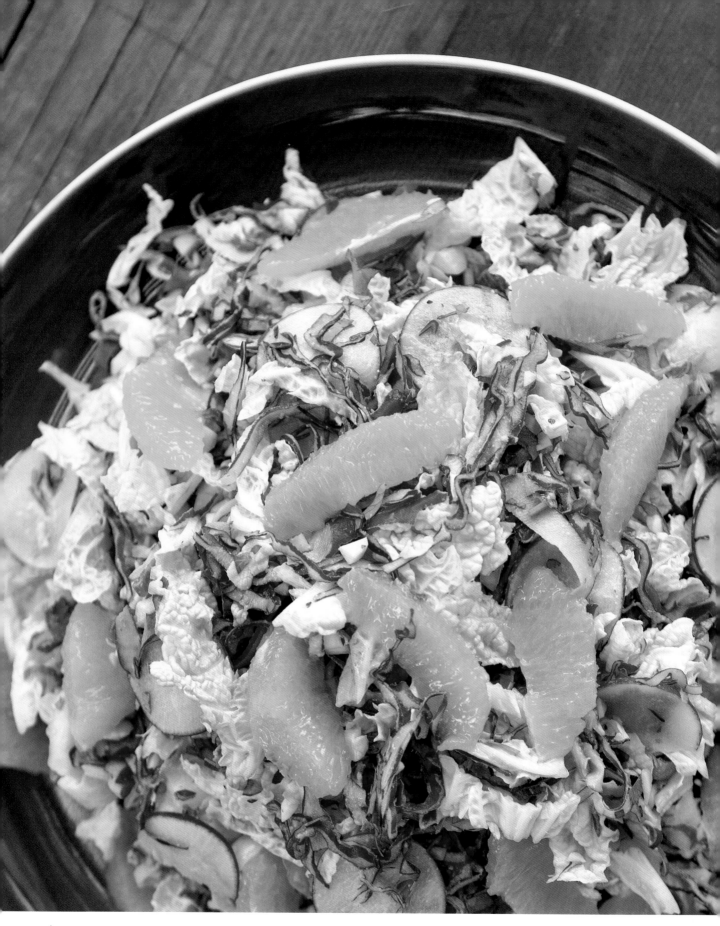

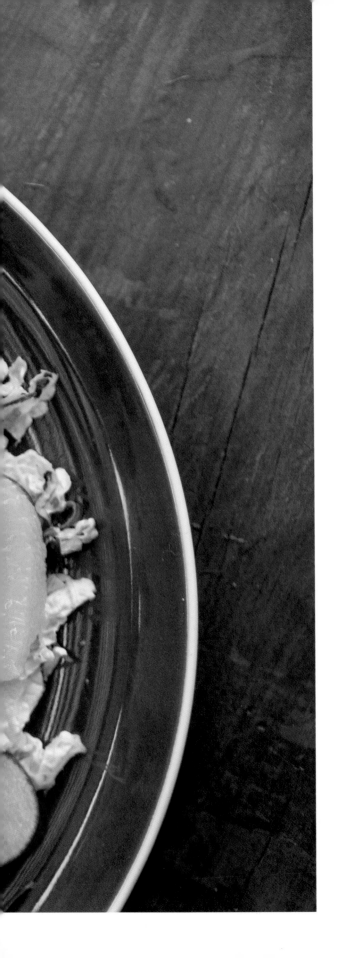

CHAPTER 4

RECIPES

DETOXIFYING JUICES

ALL JUICES YIELD AROUND 16 OUNCES (475 ML)

I like to use cucumbers and celery as the base of my juices and add apples to sweeten them. If you're sugar-sensitive, use green apples instead of red, and if you're avoiding sugar altogether, substitute the apples with additional cucumber and add a few drops of liquid stevia to taste. You can also dilute juices with purified water if they're too intense. You'll also notice I love burdock root; this is also called gobo root and can be found in Asian food markets, as well as health food stores, and is an excellent blood cleanser.

Spicy Garden
- 2 tomatoes
- 1 cucumber
- 2 to 3 stalks of celery
- 1 red bell pepper
- 1 small lime, with rind if organic
- ½ of a jalapeño or ⅛ teaspoon of cayenne pepper
- 2 cloves of garlic

Tummy Tamer
- 1 large fennel bulb with stalk
- 2 apples
- 1-inch (2.5 cm) piece of fresh ginger
- (Optional) 1 to 2 ounces (28 to 60 ml) aloe juice

Skin Glow
- 2 cucumbers
- 1 apple
- 1 red bell pepper
- 2-inch (5 cm) piece of burdock root

Root Juice
- 4 carrots
- 3 stalks of celery
- 1 apple
- ½ of a beet
- 1 to 2 radishes
- 4-inch (10 cm) piece of burdock root
- 1-inch (2.5 cm) piece of ginger

Kidney Cleanser
- 1½ cups (150 g) cranberries
- 1 cucumber
- 2 apples or pears
- Handful of watercress
- 4-inch (10 cm) piece of burdock root

Everyday Detox
- 2 cucumbers
- 3 stalks of celery
- 1 lime, with rind if organic
- Handful of spinach
- Handful of kale
- Small handful of parsley
- Small handful of cilantro
- Small handful of mint

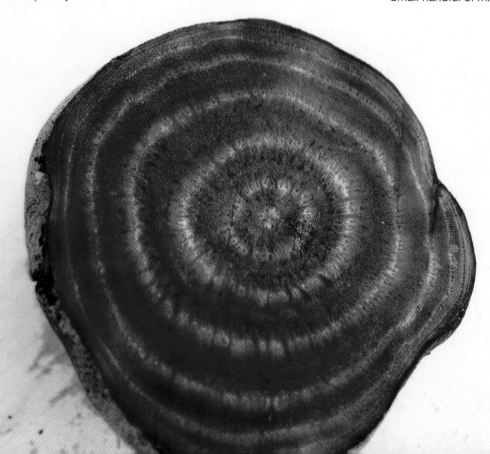

Heavy Metal Detox
- 1½ cucumbers
- 2 stalks of celery
- 1 to 2 apples
- 1 small lemon or lime, with rind if organic
- Small handful of cilantro
- Small handful of parsley
- Small handful of dandelion greens
- 1-inch (2.5 cm) piece of fresh ginger
- 1-inch (2.5 cm) piece of turmeric
- (Optional) stir in ¼ teaspoon spirulina

Blood Cleanser
- 2 apples
- 1 cucumber
- 2 kale leaves
- ½ of a lime, with rind if organic
- Small handful of mint
- 4-inch (10 cm) piece of burdock root

Red Radiance
- 2 cups (300 g) watermelon
- 1 cucumber
- 1 cup (145 g) strawberries
- Handful of mint

Liver Flush
- 1½ cucumbers
- 1 apple
- ½ of a beet
- Small handful of dandelion greens
- Small handful of parsley
- ½ of a lemon with rind, if organic
- 4-inch (10 cm) piece of burdock
- 1-inch (2.5 cm) piece of fresh ginger

Workout Recovery
- 2 cups (60 g) spinach
- 2 cups (94 g) Romaine lettuce
- 2 cups (134 g) kale, Swiss (72 g) chard, or your favorite greens
- 1½ cups (355 ml) young Thai coconut water

Juice the leafy greens and then mix with the young Thai coconut water.

SIMPLE CLEANSING TIP:
Eating a little bit of fat with your juice helps the body assimilate the fat soluble vitamins. Eat a tablespoon (14 g) of coconut oil after your juice or try blending in a small piece of avocado. This will also help sate your appetite.

CHEF TIP:
If you don't have access to a juicer, one option is to make juice with your blender by mixing in a bit of water to get the blades going and then straining it through a nut milk bag. The other option is to locate your nearest organic juice bar and pick one up on your way to work or have it delivered to your door by one of the many online juice delivery services. It's convenient, but pricy. If you choose to do a longer cleanse, you're much better off investing in a juicer.

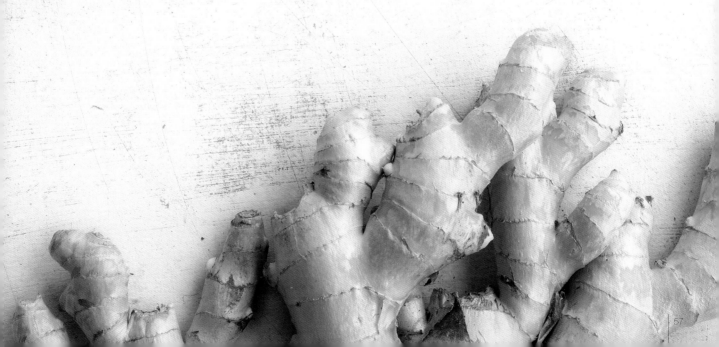

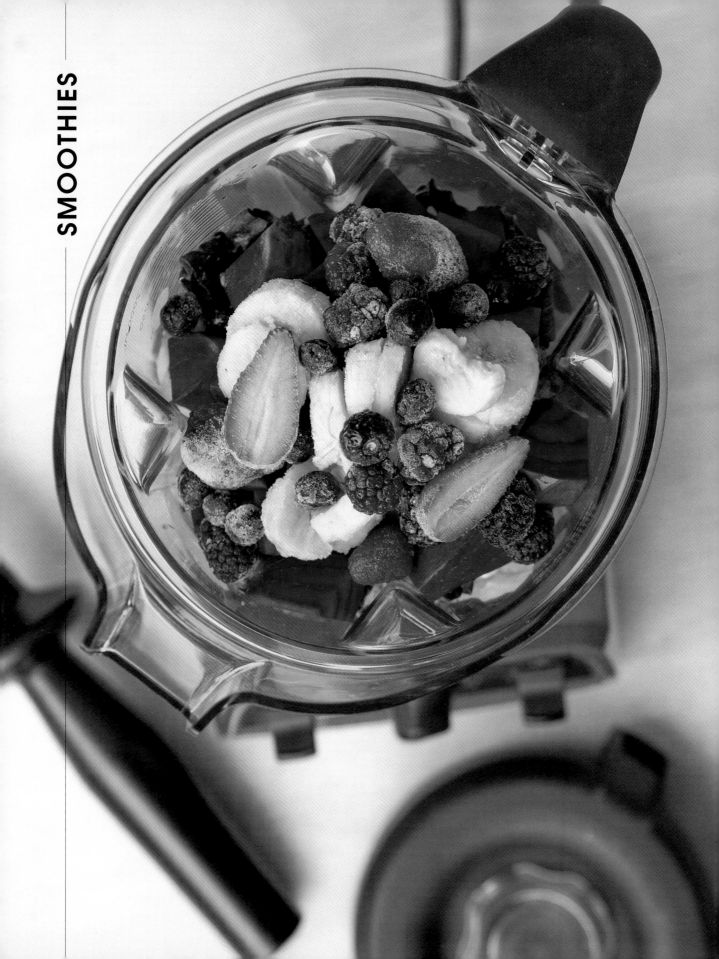

WE GOT THE BEET SMOOTHIE

There are superfoods galore in this sweet ruby-red concoction. Add more kale or other greens if you like. You'll hardly taste them beneath the creamy banana-orange flavors.

MAKES 2 SERVINGS
PREP TIME: 15 MINUTES
PLAN AHEAD: FREEZE 1 CUP (150 G) OF SLICED BANANAS.

2 medium oranges, peeled, chopped, and seeded

½ cup (120 ml) Coconut Milk (page 72), Nut Milk (page 70), or water

1 stalk celery, chopped

1 large kale leaf, chopped

1 small beet, peeled and chopped

1 cup (150 g) frozen banana chunks

½ cup (75 g) frozen mixed berries

Liquid stevia to taste

Add the items to a blender in the order listed. It's helpful to have a blender with a tamper. Put in more liquid if needed to get the blades going and blend until smooth.

PAPA-PINA DIGESTIVE ▶

This tropical delight is the perfect smoothie when things are feeling a little backed up. Papaya and pineapple both contain enzymes that are great for digestion and inflammation, while chia and flax help with regularity.

MAKES 1 TO 2 SERVINGS
PREP TIME: 15 MINUTES
PLAN AHEAD: COCONUT MILK (PAGE 72) AND COCONUT YOGURT (PAGE 168) ARE TASTY IN THIS RECIPE.

2 cups (280 g) papaya chunks

1 cup (165 g) frozen pineapple chunks

¾ cup (175 ml) Coconut Milk (page 72), Almond Milk (page 70), or young Thai coconut water

1 tablespoon (12 g) ground chia seeds

½ tablespoon ground flax seeds

¼ cup (58 g) Coconut Yogurt (page 168) or (20 g) young Thai coconut meat

Liquid stevia to taste

Process all the ingredients in a blender. Add more liquid to thin if needed.

GINGER SPICED APPLE SMOOTHIE

This smoothie reminds me of apple cobbler. Throw in some Coconut Yogurt (page 168), and you've got guilt-free dessert for breakfast.

MAKES 1 TO 2 SERVINGS
PREP TIME: 10 MINUTES
PLAN AHEAD: MAKE COCONUT MILK (PAGE 72) OR ALMOND MILK (PAGE 70).

1½ cups (355 ml) Coconut Milk (page 72) or Almond Milk (page 70)

2 cups (60 g) spinach, packed

3 red apples, chopped

3 tablespoons (45 ml) lemon juice

1 tablespoon (13 g) chia seeds

1 tablespoon (20 g) maple syrup or sweetener of choice

1½ teaspoons grated ginger

½ teaspoon cinnamon

(Optional) Dollop or two of Coconut Yogurt (page 168)

Process all ingredients in a blender until very smooth. Adjust seasonings to taste.

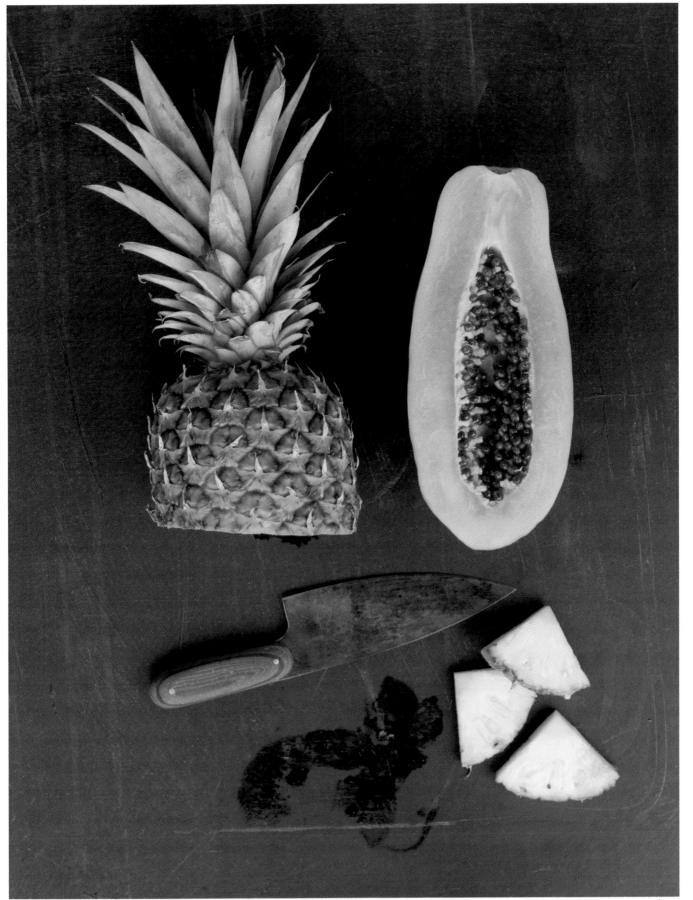

ORANGE CREAM SMOOTHIE

Who can resist the words orange cream? Orange and cucumber are lovely together and absolutely dreamy with avocado and coconut milk. This is happiness in a glass.

MAKES 2 SERVINGS
PREP TIME: 10 MINUTES
PLAN AHEAD: YOU WILL NEED ½ CUP (120 ML) COCONUT MILK (PAGE 72) OR ALMOND MILK (PAGE 70).

3 large oranges, peeled and chopped

1 cup (135 g) chopped cucumber

½ of an avocado

½ cup (120 ml) Coconut Milk (page 72) or Almond Milk (page 70)

Liquid stevia, to taste

Place all the ingredients in a blender and process until smooth.

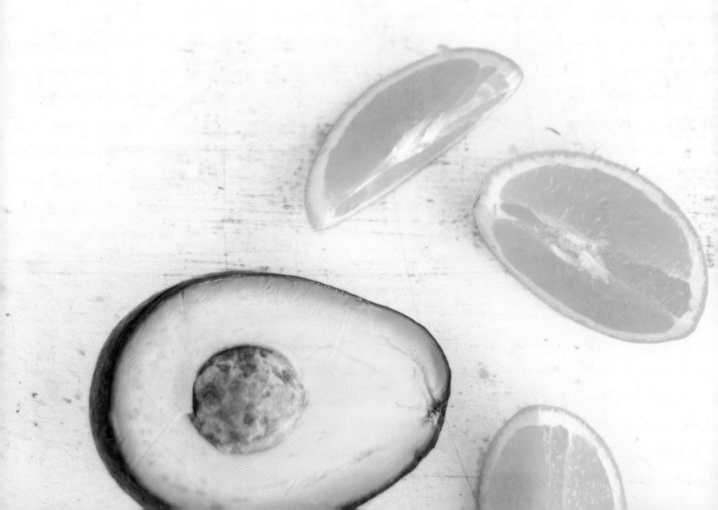

COCO GREENS

This combination of alkalizing greens with energizing coconut is a match made in health nut heaven. I practically lived off this smoothie one summer. Definitely give the strawberry variation a try as well!

MAKES 2 SERVINGS
PREP TIME: 15 MINUTES
PLAN AHEAD: (OPTIONAL) MAKE COCONUT YOGURT (PAGE 168).

2 cucumbers, chopped

2 stalks of celery, chopped

1 cup (30 g) spinach

1 cup (80 g) young Thai coconut meat or 1 cup (230 g) Coconut Yogurt (page 168)

2 tablespoons (28 ml) lime juice

1 tablespoon (14 g) coconut oil

Dash of cayenne pepper

Dash of sea salt

½ cup (70 g) ice

Run the cucumbers and celery through a juicer. Blend the juice with the remaining ingredients in a blender until smooth.

NOTE: If you don't have a juicer, blend the chopped cucumbers and celery with just enough water to get the blades going. Strain the juice through a nut milk bag.

VARIATION: For a sweet smoothie, omit the lime juice, cayenne pepper, and sea salt and add 1 cup (255 g) frozen strawberries. Sweeten with liquid stevia or your favorite sweetener to taste.

MALTED CAROB SHAKE

This is a fun, dessert-y smoothie with some sneaky spinach to pump up the nutrients. Carob powder comes from the pods of the carob tree. It's sweet and used to make chocolate-like desserts and beverages. It contains B vitamins and minerals much like chocolate, but without the stimulating effects. If you like a little kick in the pants, use raw cacao instead of carob and add a touch more sweetener.

MAKES 2 SERVINGS
PREP TIME: 10 MINUTES
PLAN AHEAD: YOU WILL NEED COCONUT MILK (PAGE 72) OR ALMOND MILK (PAGE 70) AND EITHER ⅔ CUP (153 G) COCONUT YOGURT (PAGE 168) OR (53 G) YOUNG THAI COCONUT MEAT.

⅔ cup (160 ml) Coconut Milk (page 72) or Almond Milk (page 70)

⅔ cup (153 g) Coconut Yogurt (page 168) or (53 g) young Thai coconut meat

1½ cups (45 g) loosely packed spinach

3 tablespoons (18 g) untoasted carob powder or raw cacao powder

2 tablespoons (32 g) raw almond butter

1 tablespoon (15 g) maca powder

½ tablespoon vanilla extract or dash of vanilla powder

Several drops of liquid stevia or your favorite sweetener, to taste

2 cups (280 g) ice

Place all the ingredients except for the ice in a blender and process until smooth. Add the ice and additional sweetener if needed and blend again until icy and creamy.

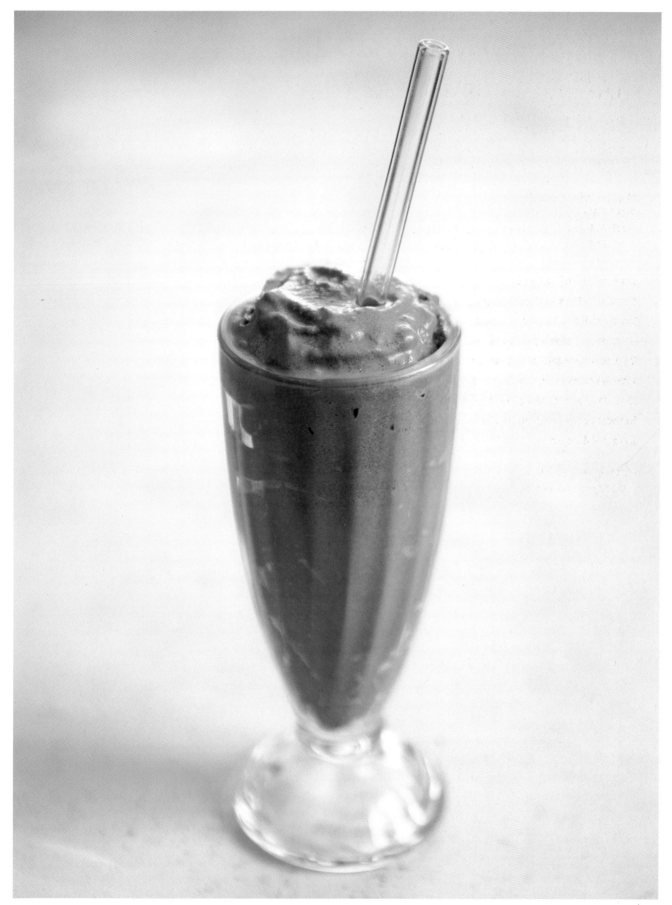

THE CALIFORNIA SMOOTHIE

Here's a fat-free fruit-and-veggie smoothie for when you want to keep it light.

MAKES 2 SERVINGS
PREP TIME: 10 MINUTES

1 large orange, peeled and chopped

½ cup (70 g) chopped cucumber

1 apple, cored and chopped

1 carrot, peeled and chopped

1 stalk of celery, chopped

Handful of spinach

3 ice cubes

A few chunks of pineapple, liquid stevia, or favorite sweetener to taste

Place all the ingredients in a blender and process until smooth.

SIMPLE SAVORY SMOOTHIE

This is not the prettiest smoothie on the block, but it's delicious nonetheless. Use more or less avocado depending on how hearty you want it and use whatever greens you have on hand. This is my go-to dinner recipe even when I'm not cleansing. It's filling but doesn't tire me out, so I'm able to be productive until bedtime.

MAKES 1 TO 2 SERVINGS
PREP TIME: 10 MINUTES

1 cup (235 ml) water

1 tomato, chopped

1 bell pepper, chopped

Handful of spinach or kale

¼ to ½ of an avocado

1 clove of garlic

Juice of half a lime

¼ teaspoon sea salt

Dash of cayenne pepper

Process all the ingredients in a blender until smooth. Adjust seasonings to taste.

HERBY VEGETABLE SMOOTHIE

Fresh and lively vegetable smoothies are a key part of my daily diet. I'll have this one for breakfast or for a light dinner many days. I often just use whatever is in the fridge, honestly. This recipe is easy to modify or substitute with other ingredients like red bell pepper, celery, or other leafy greens, or add other herbs like dill and scallions.

MAKES 1 TO 2 SERVINGS
PREP TIME: 15 MINUTES

1½ cups (355 ml) water

1 tomato, chopped

1 cucumber, chopped

1 cup (30 g) spinach

½ of an avocado

Few sprigs of basil

Few sprigs of parsley

Few sprigs of cilantro

1 to 2 cloves of garlic

Juice of one lemon or lime

Sea salt to taste

(Optional) Dash of cayenne pepper

Blend all the ingredients until smooth. Add more water to thin if needed. Adjust seasonings to taste.

CELERY-PEAR PICK-ME-UP

Think ambrosia salad in a glass, but way better. You can skip the parsley if it's too over-the-top, but I can't get enough of it. This is the perfect smoothie for those needing to keep things low-glycemic but want a creamy, sweet delight. If you have a Vitamix or high-speed blender, use ice instead of water along with the tamper. Otherwise, use water to get the blades moving.

MAKES 1 TO 2 SERVINGS
PREP TIME: 10 MINUTES

4 large stalks of celery, chopped

2 pears, chopped

1 cup (235 ml) cold water or 1½ cups (210 g) ice if you have a high-speed blender with a tamper

½ of a small avocado

(Optional) 2 to 3 sprigs of parsley

½ teaspoon cinnamon

Few drops of liquid stevia, to taste

Process all the ingredients in a blender. Add water as needed to get the blades going.

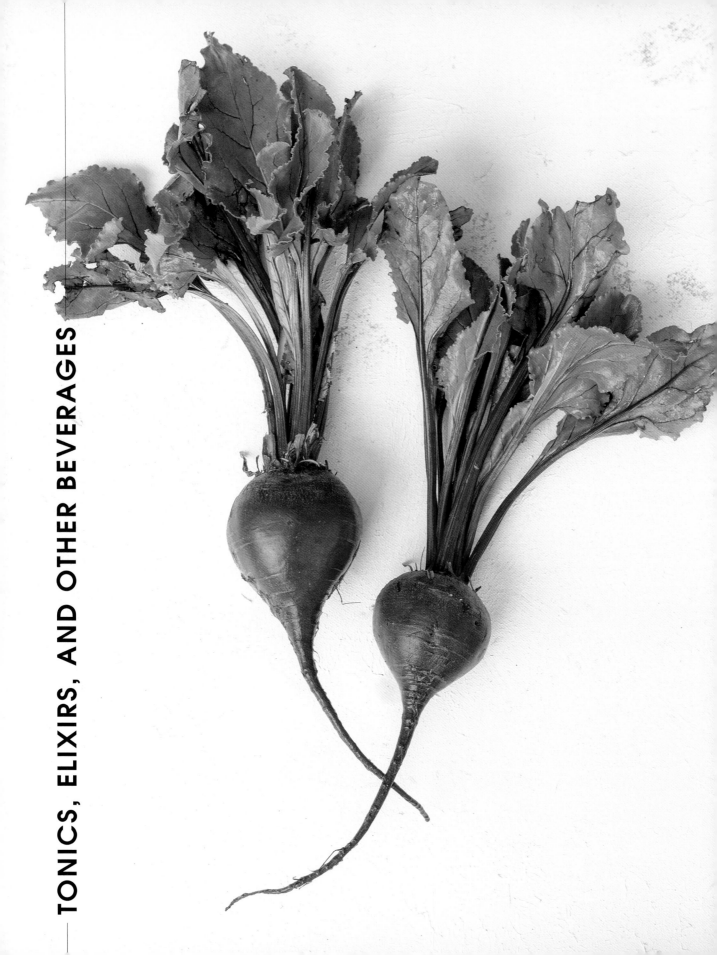

TONICS, ELIXIRS, AND OTHER BEVERAGES

BEET KVASS

Beet kvass is a traditional fermented beverage from Russia. It's an excellent liver and blood cleanser and contains enzymes and bacteria to aid digestion and food absorption. Drink 4 ounces (120 ml) with meals, upon rising, or before bed. For this recipe, you'll need a 1-quart (1 L) jar, sterilized via dishwasher or by boiling water.

MAKES 12 SERVINGS
PREP TIME: 15 MINUTES PLUS FERMENTATION TIME

½ teaspoon sea salt

1 cup (235 ml) warm water

1 medium-size beet, unpeeled

2-inch (5 cm) piece of ginger root, peeled and chopped

2-inch (5 cm) piece of turmeric root, peeled and chopped

1 clove of garlic, chopped

In a mason jar, stir together the sea salt and warm water until the salt dissolves.

Wash, but do not scrub or peel, the beet. Quarter it and then halve each section so you have 8 pieces. Add the ginger, turmeric, and garlic to the jar and then top with the chopped beet. This is to keep any pieces from floating to the top and creating mold. Fill with purified water, allowing a 2-inch (5 cm) space.

Affix the lid and place in a warm spot in the kitchen for about 5 to 7 days. Starting at day 4, taste the kvass daily until it reaches the desired tartness. It should become dark red, tart, and slightly effervescent.

It will continue to slowly ferment in the refrigerator. Use within one month.

HEALTH NOTE:
When doing wild fermentation without the use of a culture starter, you want to make sure you select freshly picked, healthy looking vegetables. Make sure your beet and other ingredients are organic and do not contain any mold.

CHEF TIP:
You can use kvass like vinegar in salad dressings, soups, and smoothies. Use the leftover fermented beets in your veggie smoothies. It's delicious!

ALMOND, NUT, OR SEED MILKS

Making your own nut milk is easier than it sounds. Once you've tried it, you'll never want to go back to the boxed stuff again. Premade nut milks often contain synthetic vitamins, carrageenan, and sugar and don't taste nearly as good as homemade nut milks. After a couple tries, you'll be able to make this in your sleep.

MAKES 4 CUPS
PREP TIME: 5 MINUTES

BASIC NUT OR SEED MILK

1 cup (145 g) raw almonds or your favorite nuts or seeds, soaked (see Note)

4 cups (946 ml) water

(Optional) 1 tablespoon (8 g) lecithin powder or granules

Process the nuts, water, and lecithin in a blender and then strain the pulp through a nylon nut milk bag.

FOR SWEETENED VANILLA NUT MILK

1 batch Basic Nut or Seed Milk

Few drops of liquid stevia, 2 to 3 Medjool dates, or 2 tablespoons (28 g) coconut nectar

1 tablespoon vanilla extract (15 ml) or ⅛ teaspoon vanilla powder

After straining out the pulp, rinse the blender container and pour the nut milk back in with sweetener and vanilla and blend again.

Store in the refrigerator for up to three days. Shake before using.

NOTE: I use unsweetened nut milk in all of the recipes in this book.
Soaking nuts make them easier to blend, but it also removes the enzyme inhibitors that make seeds and nuts dormant. These enzyme inhibitors can be very hard on the digestive system. Soaking also removes phytic acid, which can bind to zinc, iron, magnesium, calcium, chromium, and manganese in our intestinal tract. Soaking also decreases some of the acidity and bitterness, making them even more delicious. Salt or something acidic like lemon juice aids in this enzyme-removal process. Soak times are listed on the next page.

SIMPLE CLEANSING TIP: DON'T GET TOO NUTS FOR NUTS

I love nuts, but their essential fatty acid ratio is not ideal for us. We want more anti-inflammatory omega-3 than pro-inflammatory omega-6, and, sadly, nuts can throw us out of balance if we overdo it. I use a limited amount of nuts in this book, mostly as a complement to salads, and suggest using Coconut Milk (page 72) over Nut Milk whenever possible. For those suffering from acne, I noticed that when I stopped eating nuts altogether, I had less breakouts. The same thing happened to my clients and friends. Enjoy them—just don't go overboard!

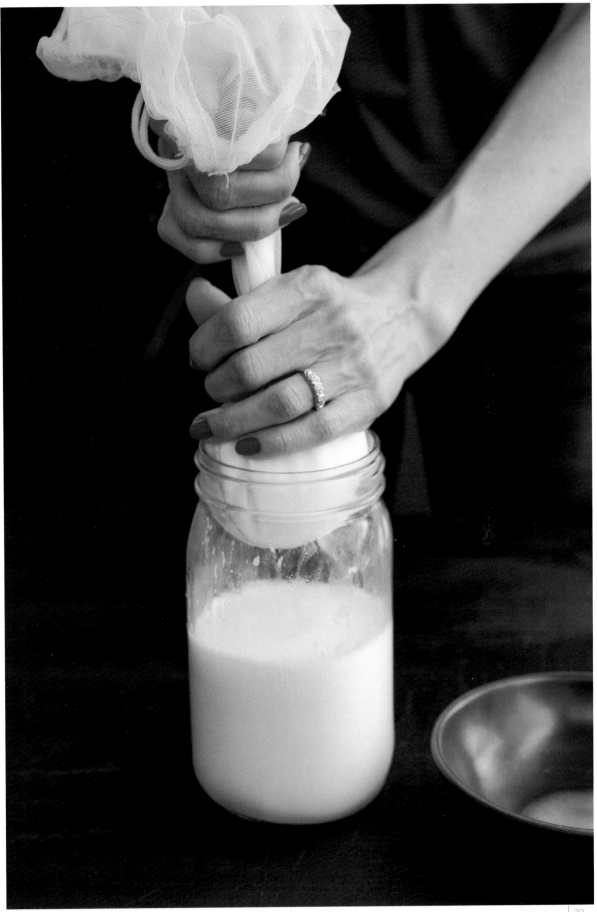

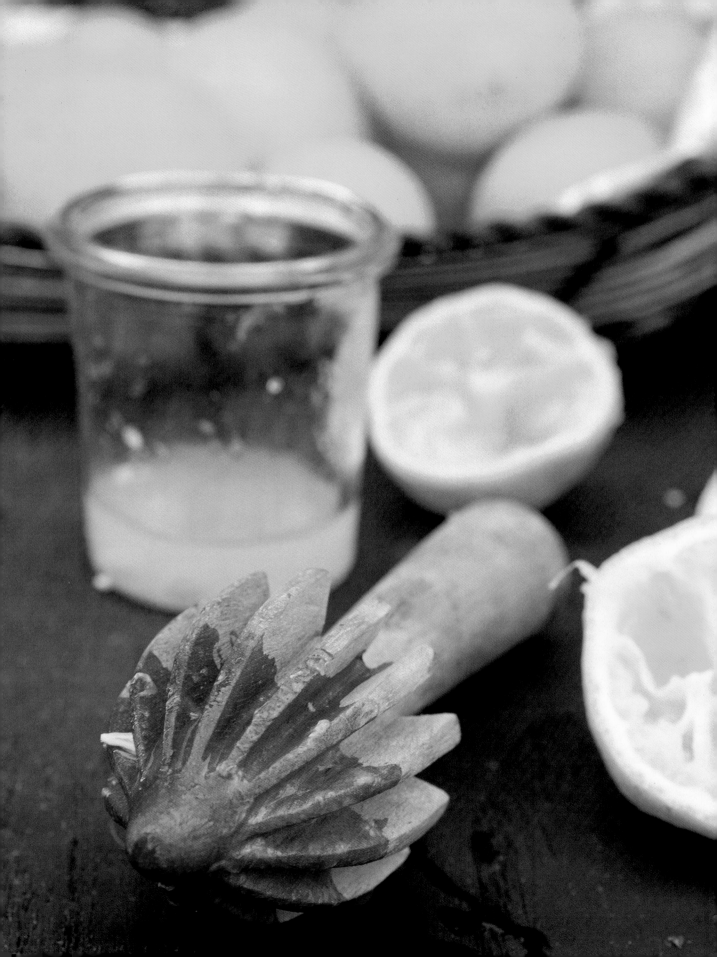

◀ LEMON WATER

Get the digestive system and the liver going first thing when you wake up with cleansing lemon juice. I recommend it even when you're not on a cleanse just to stimulate and hydrate your system. It's especially nice with hot water on chilly mornings.

MAKES 1 SERVING
PREP TIME: 5 MINUTES

1 cup (235 ml) room-temperature or hot water

Juice of 1 lemon

(Optional) Dash of cayenne pepper

(Optional) Liquid stevia, to taste

Stir all the ingredients in a glass or mug and enjoy.

SIMPLE CLEANSING TIP:
For a more potent detox drink, add ½ to 1 tablespoon (8 to 15 ml) of Bragg Apple Cider Vinegar.

GINGER-MINT LEMONADE

Start your day with this or sip it throughout the day to curb hunger while aiding digestion and adding in some minerals. It's best to use room-temperature or cool water instead of ice cold to keep your digestive fire strong.

MAKES 1 TO 2 SERVINGS
PREP TIME: 5 MINUTES

2 cups (475 ml) water

¼ cup (24 g) mint

1-inch (2.5 cm) piece of ginger, chopped

Handful of spinach

¼ cup (60 ml) or more lemon juice

Liquid stevia, to taste

Process the water, mint, ginger, and spinach in a blender and then pour through a fine sieve.

Transfer to a mason jar, add in the lemon juice, and sweeten to taste.

ADRENAL ELIXIR ▶

Stress, lack of sleep, and overconsumption of caffeine can put us into adrenal fatigue, which can create major hormonal problems. Nourish those cute little adrenals with this warming superfood blend of ashwagandha, maca, chaga mushrooms, and camu camu. They may sound strange, but they're actually traditional herbs that have been used medicinally for centuries. You can find these at most health food stores or on my website.

MAKES 1 SERVING
PREP TIME: 10 MINUTES
PLAN AHEAD: MAKE COCONUT MILK (PAGE 72) OR ALMOND MILK (PAGE 70).

1 cup (235 ml) Coconut Milk (page 72) or Almond Milk (page 70)

½ tablespoon (14 g) coconut butter or coconut oil

2 teaspoons raw carob or cacao powder

½ teaspoon maca powder

½ teaspoon freeze-dried chaga mushroom powder

¼ teaspoon camu camu

¼ teaspoon ashwaganda powder

⅛ teaspoon cinnamon

Dash of cayenne pepper

Dash of chipotle pepper

Dash of vanilla powder

Few drops of liquid stevia or your favorite sweetener

Process all the ingredients in a blender. Place the mixture in a saucepan over low heat for a few minutes until warm.

TURMERIC TONIC

This is a powerful liver tonic and anti-inflammatory that you can enjoy warm or cold. The black pepper helps make the turmeric more bioavailable to the body. A little heads up: I like my tonics strong and medicinal, but you can dilute this to whatever tastes best.

MAKES 1 SERVING
PREP TIME: 10 MINUTES

1 small lemon, rind removed

3-inch (7.5 cm) piece of turmeric root*

1-inch (2.5 cm) piece of ginger

½ cup (120 ml) or more cold or warm water

Dash of cardamom

Dash of cayenne pepper

Dash of black pepper

Few drops of liquid stevia, to taste

Run the lemon, turmeric root, and ginger through a juicer and then blend with the water, cardamom, cayenne pepper, black pepper, and liquid stevia. Dilute with additional water if too intense.

*Substitute ¼ teaspoon turmeric powder if not using fresh turmeric.

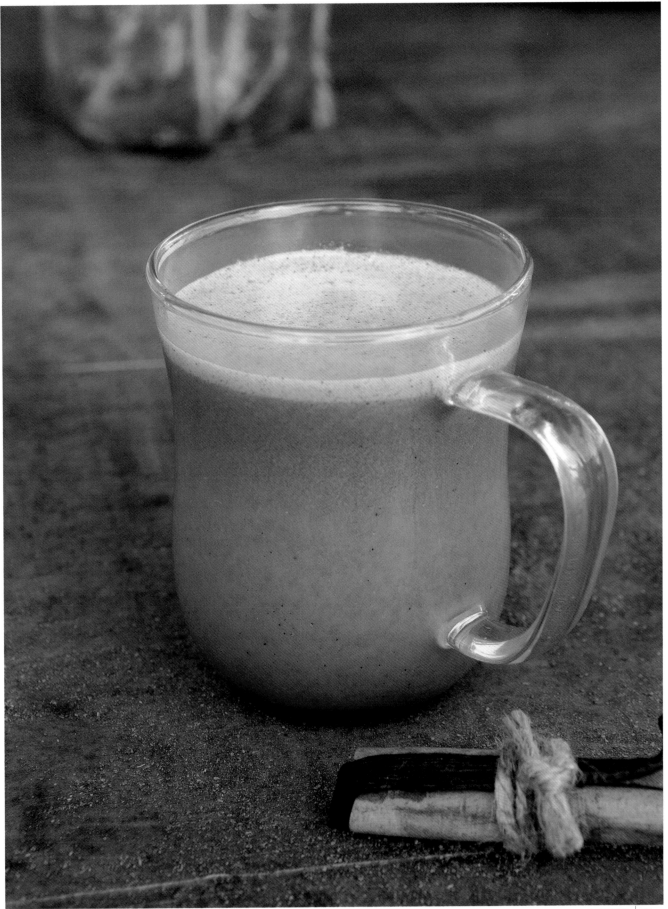

MATCHA BOOST

Matcha is a finely milled, high-quality green tea powder that contains powerful antioxidants. It provides a revitalizing lift without the side effects of coffee. My favorite brand is organic DoMatcha. They have an expensive ceremonial version and a less-pricey 2nd harvest version, which is perfect for this recipe. Enjoy it hot or cold, but keep it to one serving a day as needed.

MAKES 1 SERVING
PREP TIME: 5 MINUTES
PLAN AHEAD: MAKE COCONUT MILK (PAGE 72) OR ALMOND MILK (PAGE 70).

ICE COLD MATCHA BOOST

1 cup (235 ml) Coconut Milk (page 72) or Almond Milk (page 70)

½ cup (70 g) crushed ice

1 teaspoon matcha powder

Liquid stevia or your favorite sweetener, to taste

Place all the ingredients in a blender and process until smooth.

FOR A HOT LATTE

1 teaspon matcha powder

1 to 2 tablespoons (15 to 28 ml) hot water

1 cup (235 ml) Coconut Milk (page 72) or Almond Milk (page 70)

Liquid stevia or your favorite sweetener, to taste

Place the matcha powder and water in a mug and whisk until it turns into a smooth paste.

Separately, warm the Coconut or Almond Milk and the sweetener in a small saucepan over low heat. Use a frother to create a nice foam and then pour it over the paste and stir. You could also skip the frother and blend the warmed milk with the matcha until foamy.

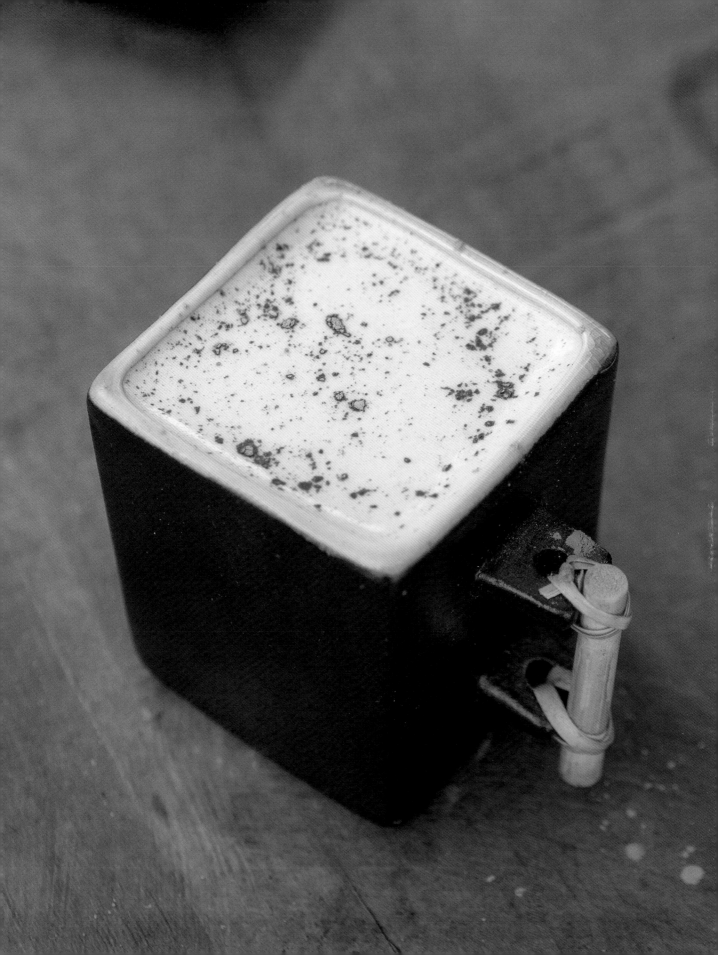

WARM TURMERIC MILK ►

I love having this soothing beverage on cold mornings and evenings. It's flavorful, but not overly spicy. It can also be enjoyed as a savory beverage, as well.

MAKES 1 SERVING
PREP TIME: 10 MINUTES
PLAN AHEAD: YOU WILL NEED 1 CUP (235 ML) COCONUT MILK (PAGE 72).

1 cup (235 ml) Coconut Milk (page 72)

½ teaspoon turmeric powder

½ teaspoon grated ginger

⅛ teaspoon garam masala*

Liquid stevia or your favorite sweetener, to taste

Warm and stir all the ingredients in a small saucepan over low heat. Pour the liquid through a fine sieve and enjoy.

*Garam masala is a popular Indian spice blend of black pepper, cardamom, cinnamon, cloves, cumin, and coriander.

COLD BUSTER

Besides being an amazing detox tonic, this is a great alternative if you feel a cold or flu coming on and don't want to take liver-toxic over-the-counter cold meds. It's very potent and can be taken as often as needed.

MAKES 1 SERVING
PREP TIME: 10 MINUTES

1 lemon

2-inch (5 cm) piece of ginger

2 cloves of garlic

½ cup (120 ml) or more purified hot water

Few drops of liquid stevia or raw honey

1 drop oil of oregano

Dash of cayenne pepper

Juice the lemon, ginger, and garlic. Mix with the hot water, sweetener, oregano oil, and cayenne.

Dilute with additional water if too intense. Sip slowly.

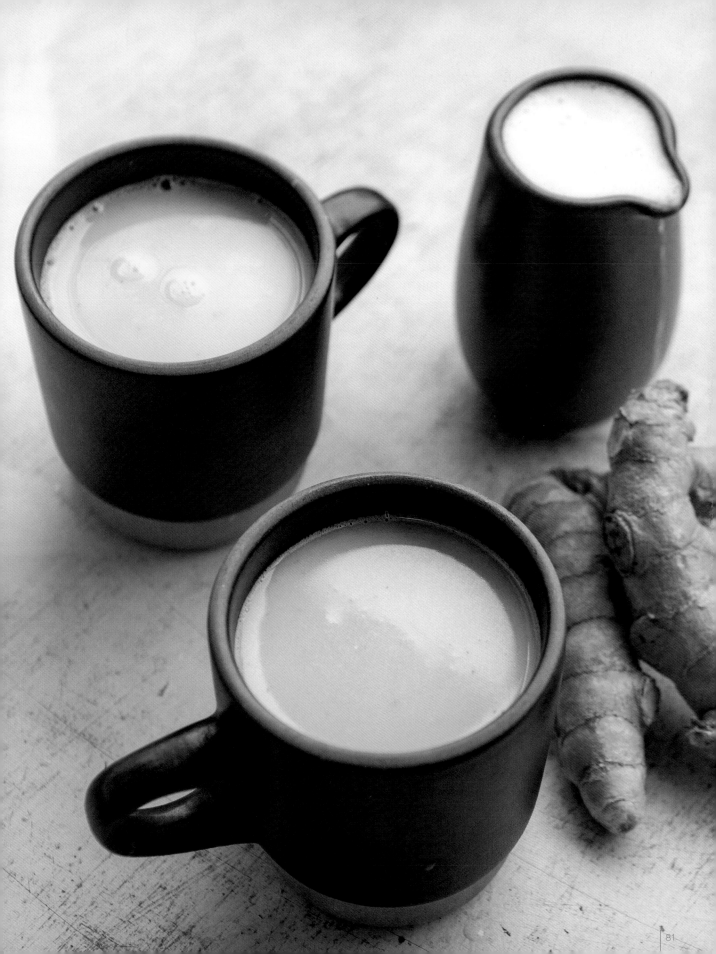

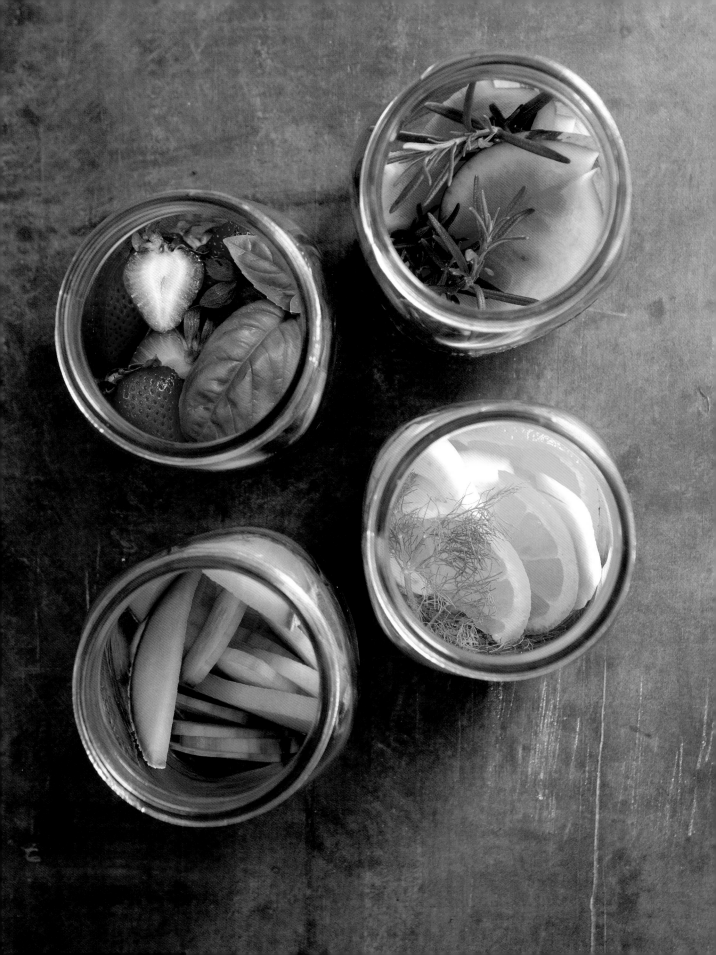

FRUIT-INFUSED WATER

We need to get enough water each day somehow, so why not spruce it up with some fruits, veggies, and herbs. Below are my favorite combinations, but I'm sure you can come up with at least a dozen other ones. I usually refresh each batch several times before discarding. If you're making this for more than just yourself, use a 2-quart (2 L) jar and double the quantities.

MAKES 2 SERVINGS
PREP TIME: 5 MINUTES PLUS A HALF HOUR
OR MORE FOR FLAVORS TO MINGLE

Place all the ingredients for your chosen infusion in a 1-quart (1 L) mason jar. If using herbs, bruise or muddle them first with a wooden spoon. Fill the jar with filtered water and allow at least half an hour for the flavors to release—but the longer you leave it, the better it tastes. Sweeten to taste with liquid stevia if desired.

When you refill your jar with water, muddle the contents with a spoon to release more flavor.

STRAWBERRY-BASIL
1 cup (170 g) sliced strawberries

½ cup (20 g) loosely packed fresh basil

CUCUMBER-MINT
1 cup (119 g) cucumber, sliced

½ cup (48 g) fresh mint

WATERMELON-ROSEMARY
2 cups (300 g) watermelon, cubed

1 sprig of rosemary

CANTALOUPE-CUCUMBER
1 cup (160 g) cantaloupe, sliced

½ of a cucumber, sliced

ORANGE FENNEL
1 small orange, sliced

1 cup (87 g) chopped fennel

RASPBERRY KOMBUCHA MARGARITA

Kombucha is an effervescent, fermented tea that aids digestion, boosts the immune system, and supports liver detoxification. Drink it straight-up before meals to enhance digestion or try it in this recipe for a fun and refreshing mocktail.

MAKES 1 SERVING
PREP TIME: 10 MINUTES

⅔ cup (160 ml) kombucha

⅓ cup fresh or frozen (42 or 83 g) raspberries, thawed

5 small leaves of fresh mint

1 tablespoon (15 ml) lime juice

½ teaspoon grated ginger

½ cup (70 g) or more crushed ice

Liquid stevia, to taste

Place all the ingredients in a blender and process until blended. Add more ice if you prefer a more slushy version.

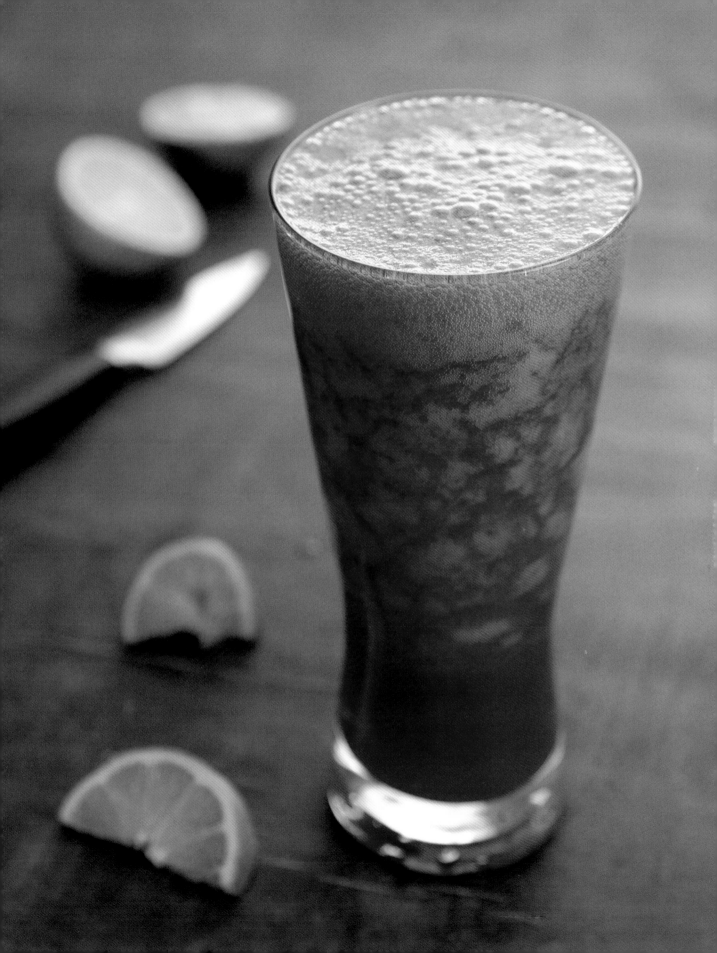

CHIA SEED BEVERAGES

I love those fruity chia drinks you find in the health food stores, but they can be really pricey. I prefer to make my own for a fraction of the cost. Here are three chia drinks that I love, but I'm sure you could come up plenty of your own. Almost any juice or liquid works well. I've even made chia drinks with chilled rooibos and green tea.

PLAN AHEAD: YOU WILL NEED ½ CUP (110 G) OR MORE OF CHIA GEL (OPPOSITE)

GRAPEFRUIT-GINGER CHIA DRINK

MAKES 1 SERVING

½ cup (110 g) chia gel

½ cup (120 g) fresh-squeezed grapefruit juice

¼ teaspoon or more ginger juice*

Liquid stevia to taste

Stir all the ingredients in a glass until combined.

*If you don't own a juicer, grate the ginger and then squeeze it through a nut milk bag or fine sieve.

CHIA FRESCA

MAKES 1 TO 2 SERVINGS

1 cup (235 ml) cold water

½ cup (110 g) chia gel

Juice of ½ a lemon or lime

Liquid stevia to taste

Stir all the ingredients together in a glass until combined.

STRAWBERRIES AND CREAM CHIA DRINK

MAKES 1 SERVING

⅔ cup (160 ml) Almond Milk (page 70) or Coconut Milk (page 72)

⅓ cup (48 g) strawberries

⅓ cup (73 g) chia gel

Dash of vanilla powder or ¼ teaspoon vanilla extract

Liquid stevia to taste

Blend the milk and strawberries until very smooth. Transfer to a glass and stir in the Chia Gel.

CHIA GEL

This simple gel is a great addition to smoothies and soups when you want to add some thickness as well as some extra essential fatty acids and protein.

MAKES ABOUT 3 CUPS (660 G)
PREP TIME: 10 MINUTES PLUS 6 TO 8 HOURS TO SET

2 cups (475 ml) water

⅓ cup (69 g) chia seeds

Mix the chia seeds and water in a mason jar and allow to sit for 5 minutes. Mix it again to remove any lumps and allow it to sit for 6 to 8 hours or overnight in the refrigerator.

This will last 7 days in the refrigerator.

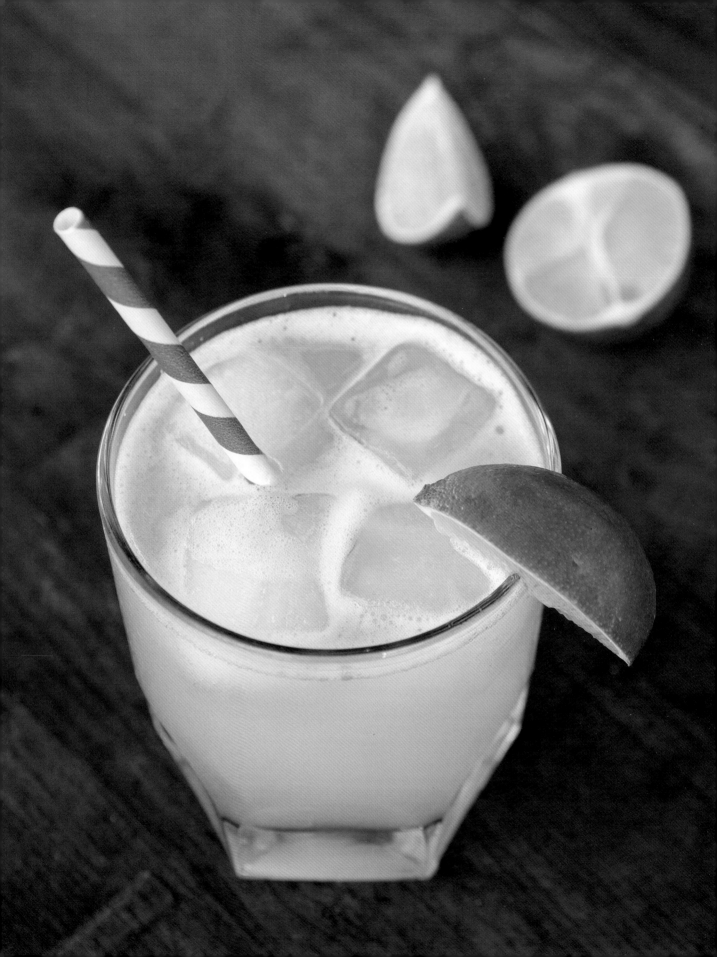

ELECTROLYTE LIMEADE

This is a great post-workout drink. Coconut water replenishes electrolytes while methylsulfonylmethane, or MSM, helps recovery. MSM is a natural sulfur supplement that reduces inflammation and is essential for the body to create glutathione, which is important for detoxification. MSM has been found to be beneficial for bones, joints, skin, hair, and nails, so consider this a little beauty tonic, as well.

MAKES 1 TO 2 SERVINGS
PREP TIME: 5 MINUTES

1 cup (235 ml) young Thai coconut water

2 tablespoons (28 ml) lime juice

(Optional) Pinch of MSM crystals

Dash of sea salt

Liquid stevia, to taste

Stir or blend all the ingredients together and serve over ice.

HEALTH NOTE: *Coconut water is an excellent source of electrolytes and outperforms commercial sport drinks when it comes to post-exercise rehydration. The high potassium content is helpful in lowering high blood pressure and increasing circulation, which may reduce the risk of stroke and cardiovascular disease.*

SOUPS

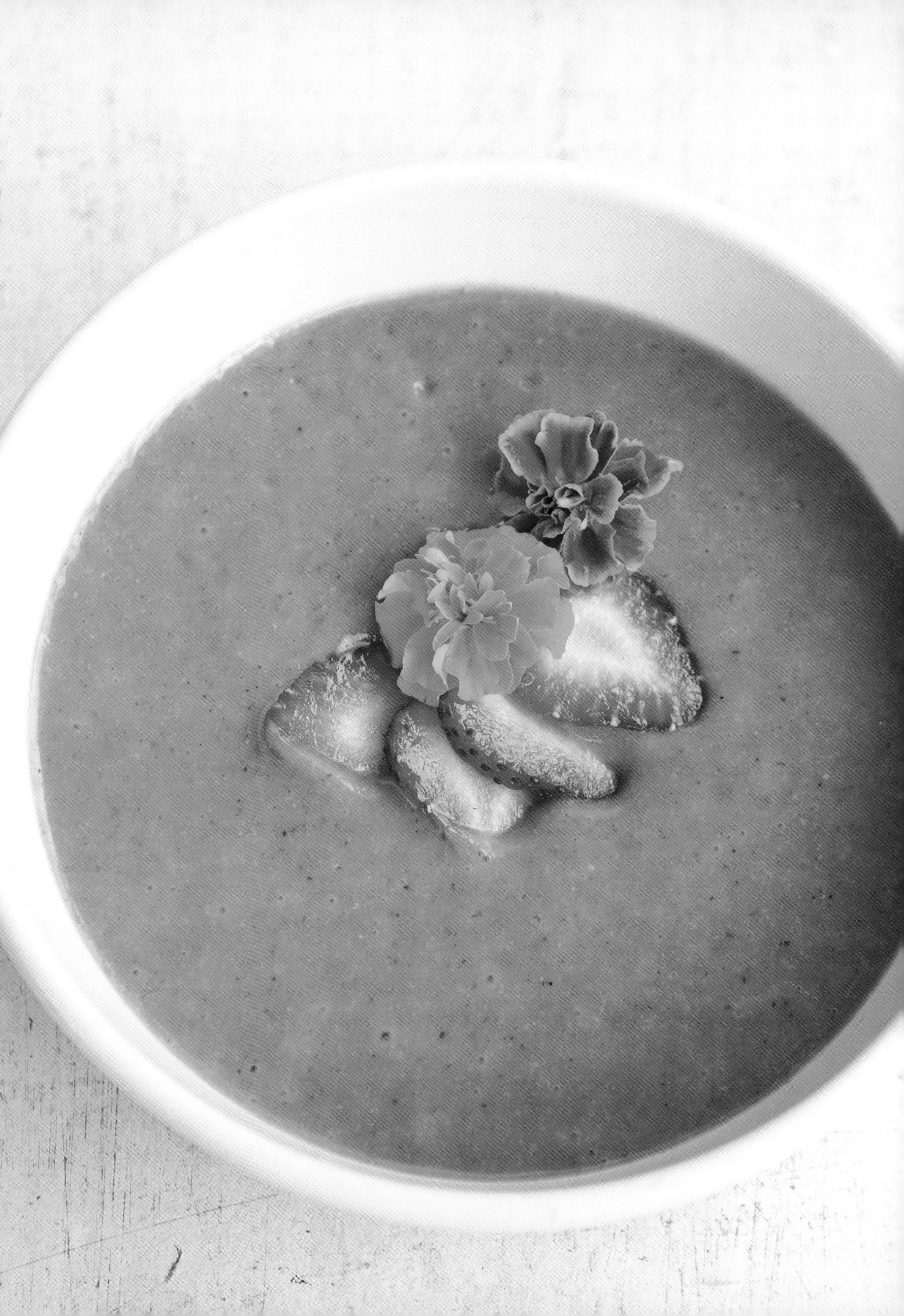

◀ SAVORY STRAWBERRY SOUP

This unconventional soup is a bit like a strawberry gazpacho. It's the right balance of savory and sweet, with undertones of basil and mint. It's perfect when you're in the mood for something different.

MAKES 2 TO 3 SERVINGS
PREP TIME: 30 MINUTES

3 cups chopped fresh or frozen (435 g or 765 g) strawberries, thawed

1 cup (235 ml) coconut water

⅔ cup (53 g) young Thai coconut meat or Coconut Yogurt (page 168)

2 tablespoons (5 g) chopped basil

2 tablespoons (12 g) chopped mint

1 tablespoon (15 ml) coconut aminos

½ teaspoon lime zest

Dash of cayenne pepper, to taste

Dash of black pepper, to taste

Blend all the ingredients until very smooth. Adjust seasonings to taste. Serve chilled or at room temperature. It's extra nice with a dollop of Cashew Sour Cream (page 98). If desired, you can garnish with edible flowers and additional chopped strawberries.

CUCUMBER-MINT SOUP

This is a variation of the Beauty Soup from my first book, Going Raw. *Just think how great your skin is going to look while enjoying this light and creamy soup. The yield says two servings, but I'm pretty sure you can finish it in one sitting. For a more filling soup or if you want some texture, add some diced tomatoes and sweet onions at the end before serving.*

MAKES 2 SERVINGS
PREP TIME: 10 MINUTES

1½ cups (355 ml) water, Coconut Milk (page 72) or Almond Milk (page 70)

1½ cups (205 g) chopped cucumber (about 1 cucumber)

1 small avocado

⅓ cup (32 g) fresh mint

2 tablespoons (28 ml) lime or lemon juice

1 clove of garlic

½ teaspoon sea salt or to taste

Dash of cayenne or chipotle pepper

Dash of fresh black pepper

(Optional) ⅛ teaspoon or more spirulina

Add all the ingredients to a blender and process until smooth.

SWEET PEA, MINT, AND FENNEL SOUP

Fresh peas are one legume, besides green beans, I can make an exception for when cleansing. They are easy to digest for most people and contain a powerhouse of nutrients like vitamin K for strong bones and healthy blood clotting, lutein for eye health, vitamin C, B vitamins, iron, magnesium, and protein. The fennel and mint brighten up the flavor of this delectable soup, which can be enjoyed chilled or warmed.

MAKES 2 SERVINGS
PREP TIME: 15 MINUTES
PLAN AHEAD: YOU WILL NEED 1½ CUPS (355 ML) COCONUT MILK (PAGE 72) OR ALMOND MILK (PAGE 70).

SOUP BASE

1½ cups (355 ml) Coconut Milk (page 67) or Almond Milk (page 65)

1 cup fresh or frozen (150 g or 130 g) peas, thawed

½ cup (44 g) chopped fennel

1 zucchini, peeled and chopped

¼ cup mint (24 g), loosely packed

2 tablespoons (28 ml) lemon juice

1 to 2 Medjool dates, pitted

1 tablespoon (10 g) chopped shallot

Salt and pepper to taste

ADDITIONAL

½ bulb of fennel, shaved

½ cup (75 g) peas

Process all the ingredients in a blender until smooth. Adjust seasonings to taste. Pour into serving bowls and top with additional peas and thinly shaved fennel. Add more if you like your soup chunky.

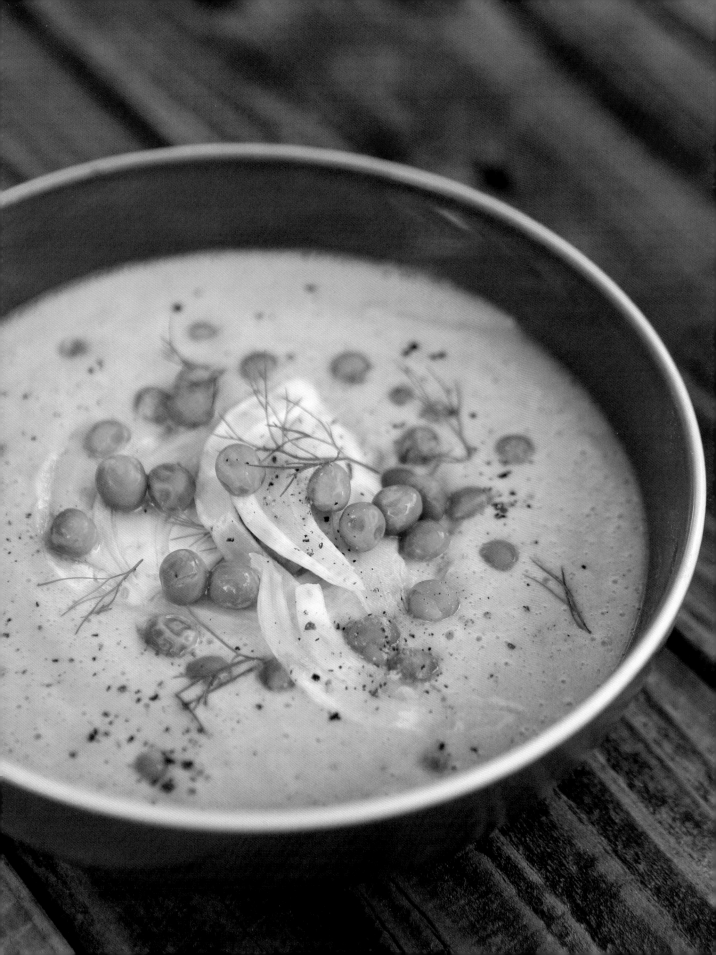

SOPA VERDE

Visually, this Mexican-style green soup might not inspire you, but if you just close your eyes and let your taste buds do their thing, you will find yourself in flavor country. Adapt this recipe to your liking. You can switch up the base using different peppers like ancho or hatch chilis, or add in some cumin and oregano for an even richer flavor.

MAKES 2 SERVINGS
PREP TIME: 20 MINUTES

SOUP BASE

3 tomatoes, chopped

½ of a cucumber, chopped

2 stalks of celery, chopped

2 cups (60 g) loosely packed spinach

Juice of one lime

2 tablespoons (20 g) chopped sweet yellow onion

Few sprigs of cilantro

Small piece of jalapeño, seeded

1 tablespoon (14 g) coconut nectar or your favorite sweetener (optional, for flavor balance)

½ teaspoon sea salt

⅛ teaspoon chipotle pepper

ADD-INS

1 tomato, diced

1 small avocado, cubed

½ of a cucumber, diced

Kernels from one ear of fresh organic corn (optional; omit if allergic to corn)

Dollop of Cashew Sour Cream (page 98)

Place all the soup base ingredients in a blender in the order listed. Blend on low to medium speed until smooth. Adjust seasonings to taste.

Pour into serving bowls and top with any of the add-ins.

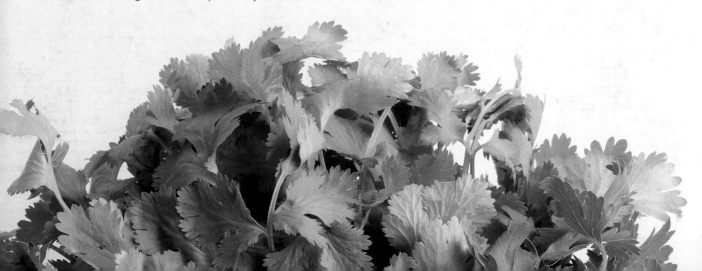

CREAM OF TOMATO SOUP

This slightly sweet and creamy soup is great served chilled in the summer or gently warmed for a cold, rainy day. Tomatoes contain lycopene, a powerful phytonutrient and antioxidant. Blending them in a high-power blender increases their bioavailability.

MAKES 2 TO 3 SERVINGS
PREP TIME: 15 MINUTES

4 Roma tomatoes, seeded and chopped

2 cups (475 ml) water

½ of an avocado

⅓ cup (13 g) fresh basil

2 to 3 tablespoons (28 to 42 g) coconut nectar or 2 large Medjool dates, pitted

2 cloves of garlic

1 teaspoon dried oregano

1 teaspoon sea salt, or to taste

Blend all the ingredients until smooth. Pour into serving bowls and top with fresh cracked pepper and a drizzle of olive oil or Cashew Sour Cream (page 98).

COCONUT-BROCCOLI SHORBA

Curry with coconut milk is my favorite Indian food flavor combo. Enjoy this one cold or warmed gently on the stovetop. You can vary the soup by trying different curry blends, as some are more floral while some are spicier. Try to avoid blends with added salt or adjust seasonings to taste so that you don't over season.

MAKES 2 TO 3 SERVINGS
PREP TIME: 20 MINUTES
PLAN AHEAD: MAKE COCONUT MILK (PAGE 72).

3 cups (700 ml) Coconut Milk (page 72)

1 cup (71 g) broccoli florets, chopped

2 teaspoons curry powder

½ of an avocado

2 to 3 Medjool dates, pitted

2 tablespoons (28 ml) lime juice

3-inch (7.5 cm) piece of fresh turmeric root or 2 teaspoons dried powder

2 teaspoons grated ginger

1 small clove of garlic

½ teaspoon sea salt

Process all the ingredients in a blender until smooth. Adjust seasonings to taste. Garnish with some additional chopped broccoli florets for a little color and texture.

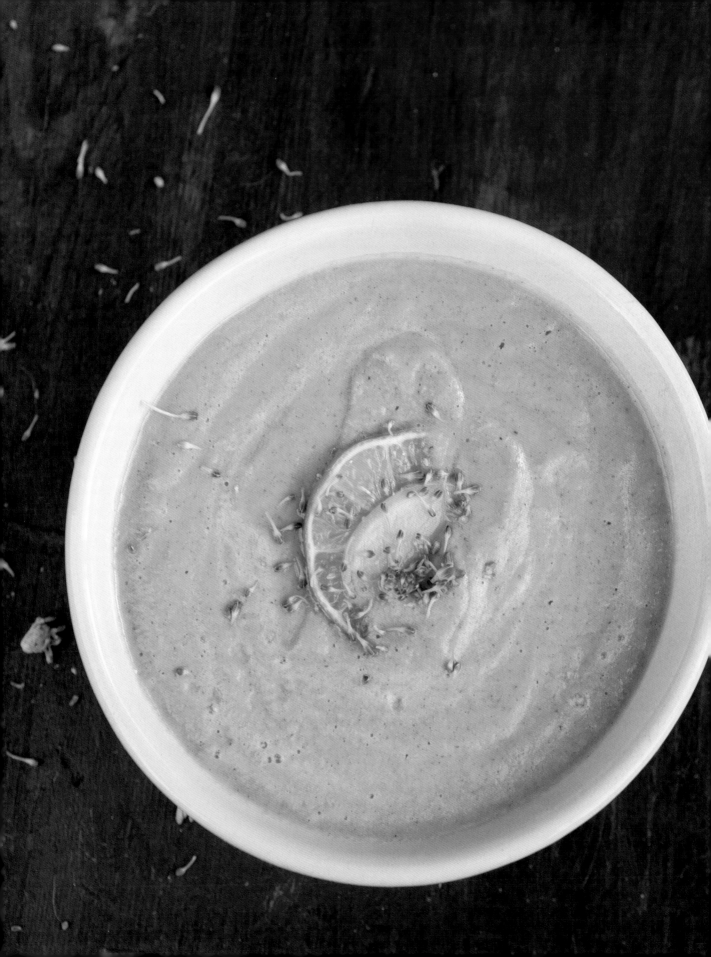

DILLY BEET SOUP ▶

This version of a creamy borscht takes me back to my Eastern European roots. I grew up eating this soup and now have a way to enjoy it in a snap. It's great chilled or gently warmed.

MAKES 2 TO 3 SERVINGS
PREP TIME: 15 MINUTES

SOUP BASE

2½ cups (570 ml) water

1 cup (225 g) chopped beets

2 stalks of celery

¼ of a medium avocado

3 tablespoons (45 ml) lemon juice

1 to 2 Medjool dates, pitted

Few sprigs of dill

1 clove of garlic

½ teaspoon sea salt

ADDITIONAL

Avocado, cubed

Cashew Sour Cream

Process all the ingredients in a blender until smooth. Adjust seasonings to taste. Pour into serving bowls and top with cubed avocado and a dallop of Cashew Sour Cream (see below).

CASHEW SOUR CREAM

MAKES 8 SERVINGS
PREP TIME: 5 MINUTES
PLAN AHEAD: SOAK 1 CUP OF CASHEWS FOR 2 HOURS

1 cup (67.5 g) cashews, soaked

½ cup (120 ml) water

2 tablespoons (30 ml) lemon juice

Process all ingredients in a blender until very smooth. Add more lemon juice if you like it tart. Chill to firm. Cashew Sour Cream will keep in the refrigerator for one week.

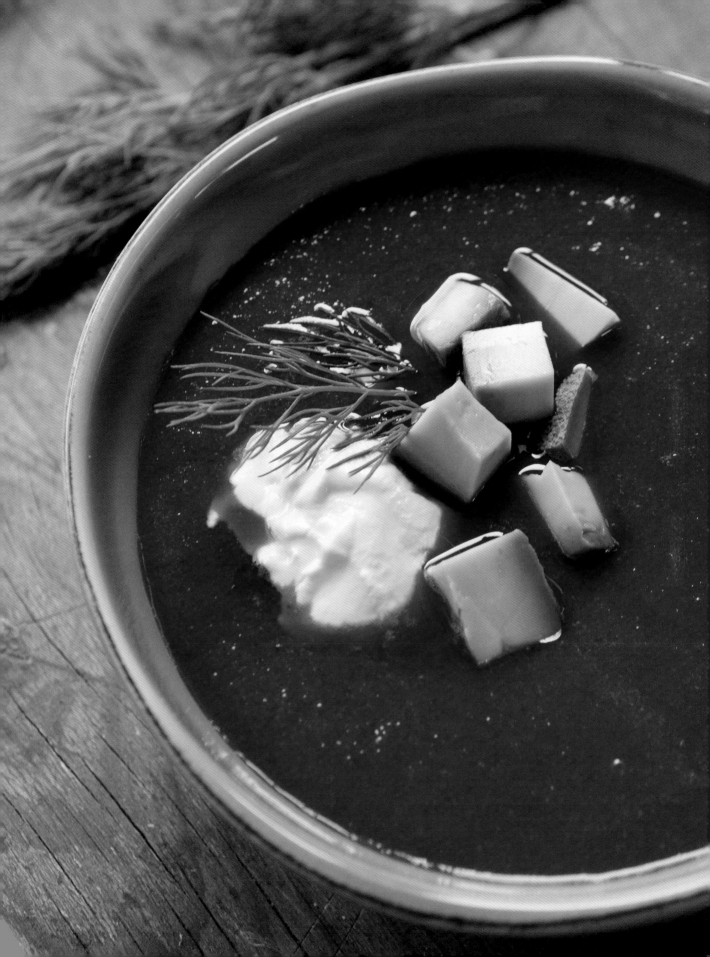

CURRIED SEAWEED SOUP

I like to sip on this nourishing soup in a mug or Thermos during the cooler months. It's rich in natural iodine, which is essential for every cell in the body. Because iodine is found almost exclusively in ocean vegetables and seafood, the majority of the world's population is actually deficient. Kelp and kombu (a variety of kelp) contain the highest amounts of iodine, but should be enjoyed in moderation if you have Hashimoto's thyroiditis or Graves' disease, both autoimmune diseases of the thyroid, as high doses could worsen symptoms.

MAKES 3 TO 4 SERVINGS
PREP TIME: 20 MINUTES

SEAWEED

⅔ cup (24 g) loosely packed dried wild Atlantic kombu

¾ cup (175 ml) hot water

SOUP BASE

2½ cups (570 ml) warm or room-temperature water

3 tablespoons (32 g) chickpea miso

2 tablespoons (24 g) coconut oil

1½ tablespoons (23 ml) lemon juice

1 tablespoon (6 g) curry powder

1 tablespoon (8 g) grated ginger

1 to 2 Medjool dates, pitted

FOR THE SEAWEED

Place the dried kombu in a small bowl with ¾ cup (175 ml) hot water and allow to soak for 20 minutes. Reserve the soaking liquid.

FOR THE SOUP

Blend all the ingredients in the Soup Base, as well as the kombu and soaking liquid, in a blender until smooth. Adjust seasonings. This tastes best warmed gently over the stovetop. The soup keeps for 3 days in the refrigerator.

SIMPLE CLEANSING TIP:
I recommend Atlantic sea vegetables over Pacific varieties since there is concern over possible contamination due to the Japanese nuclear fallout.

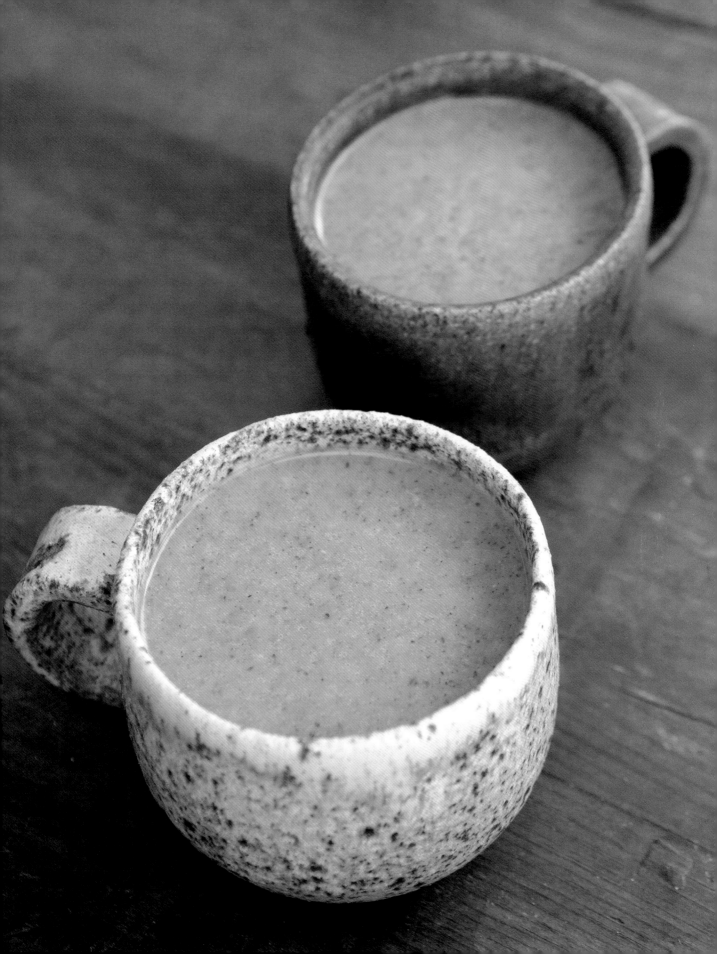

SUPER GREENS COCONUT SOUP (COOKED)

This is a great soup when you need warming foods, especially if you are cleansing during the cooler months. It's very grounding and nourishing and ideal for those who can't eat raw cruciferous greens.

MAKES 2 SERVINGS
PREP TIME: 30 MINUTES
PLAN AHEAD: MAKE COCONUT MILK (PAGE 72).

1 tablespoon (14 g) coconut oil

½ of a sweet or yellow onion, diced

2 cloves of garlic, crushed

5 cups (275 g) chopped greens like kale, chard, collards, or beet greens or a mix of all

3 cups (700 ml) Coconut Milk (page 72)

1 tablespoon (14 g) coconut nectar

Juice of one small lime

Dash of cayenne pepper

Salt and pepper to taste

Heat the oil in a pot on medium to medium-low heat and add in the onion. Stirring regularly, cook until the onion becomes translucent and softened. Add the garlic and stir until it becomes fragrant.

Add the greens and cook for three to five minutes until wilted.

Pour in the coconut milk, coconut nectar, lime juice, cayenne pepper, salt, and pepper and bring to a simmer. Use an immersion blender to purée the ingredients, or you can transfer to a blender in small batches.

Adjust seasonings to taste and serve.

VEGETABLE SOUP (COOKED)

This is an easy and nourishing soup for a winter cleanse. Kombu adds iodine and trace minerals while giving it a deeper flavor. Get creative and try other vegetables that are native to where you live. Parsnips are a great substitute for carrots, potatoes are very grounding if you want to slow your cleanse a bit, and herbs can give this soup more dimension. Herbamare is a nice addition, or spice it up with some cayenne pepper or hot sauce.

MAKES 4 SERVINGS
PREP TIME: 30 MINUTES PLUS 1 HOUR TO SIMMER

2 quarts (2 L) water

½ a head medium-size green cabbage, chopped

4 carrots, peeled and chopped

2 stalks of celery, chopped

1 medium sweet onion, diced

4 cloves of garlic, chopped

Few sprigs of parsley, chopped

2-inch-by-6-inch (5 cm-by-15 cm) strip of kombu

1 bay leaf

1 teaspoon sea salt or to taste

Freshly ground pepper to taste

Place all the ingredients in a large pot and bring to boil. Reduce the heat and simmer uncovered for sixty minutes. Remove the kombu, chop into little pieces, and return to the soup. Remove the bay leaf and serve.

Store leftovers in the refrigerator for 2 days.

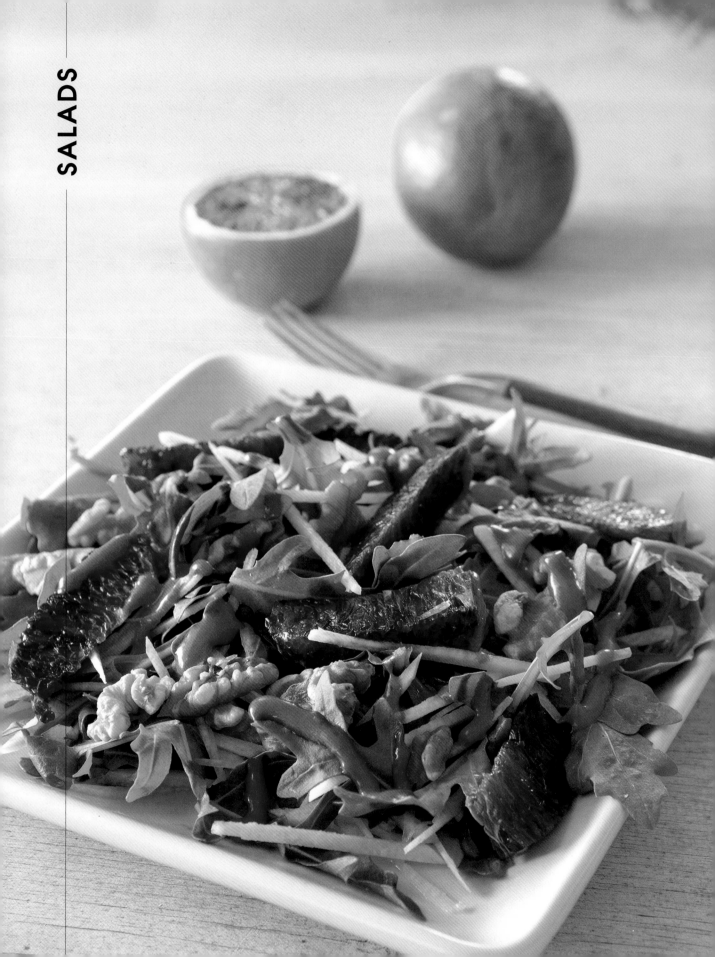

ARUGULA SALAD WITH JICAMA, BLOOD ORANGE, AND RASPBERRY VINAIGRETTE

This sweet, tart, and crunchy salad is almost too pretty to eat. It goes well with a savory soup like Cream of Tomato (page 95) or Cucumber-Mint (page 91).

MAKES 2 TO 3 SERVINGS
PREP TIME: 20 MINUTES
PLAN AHEAD: SOAK RAW WALNUTS FOR 4 TO 6 HOURS, RINSE, AND DRAIN.

RASPBERRY VINAIGRETTE DRESSING

1 cup fresh or frozen (125 g or 250 g) raspberries, thawed if necessary

¼ cup (60 ml) olive oil

2 tablespoons (28 ml) lemon juice

2 tablespoons (40 g) raw honey or coconut nectar

3 to 4 leaves basil, chopped

SALAD

3 cups (60 g) arugula, loosely packed

2 cups (260 g) julienned jicama

⅓ cup (40 g) raw walnuts, soaked and chopped

3 blood oranges or regular oranges, supremed

FOR THE DRESSING

Blend all the dressing ingredients until smooth.

FOR THE SALAD

Toss the salad ingredients in a large bowl and then drizzle with the dressing.

CHEF TIP:

"Supreme" is the culinary term for removing the rind, pith, membrane, and seeds of citrus fruits.

CARROT RIBBON SALAD

Colorful heirloom carrots are only available a few weeks out of the year. If you don't have them at your local farmer's market, then by all means grab those vibrant orange ones and make yourself one of the tastiest salads you'll ever eat. The sweet carrots with bitter arugula and fresh herbs will make your taste buds sing!

MAKES 4 SERVINGS
PREP TIME: 30 MINUTES

SALAD

3 to 4 large heirloom carrots

3 cups (60 g) packed wild or baby arugula

¼ cup (35 g) raw pine nuts

FRESH HERB DRESSING

⅓ cup (80 ml) olive oil

¼ cup (60 ml) lemon juice

2 tablespoons (6 g) fresh, finely chopped chives

2 tablespoons (6 g) fresh, finely chopped basil

2 teaspoons raw honey or coconut nectar

2 teaspoons whole grain Dijon mustard

Sea salt and ground pepper to taste

FOR THE SALAD

Use a peeler to make long carrot ribbons—you will want about 3 cups (366 g) of carrots when you're done. In a large bowl, toss the carrots, arugula, and pine nuts together.

FOR THE DRESSING

Quickly pulse the ingredients in a mini blender or whisk in a bowl. Pour over the salad, mix well, and serve.

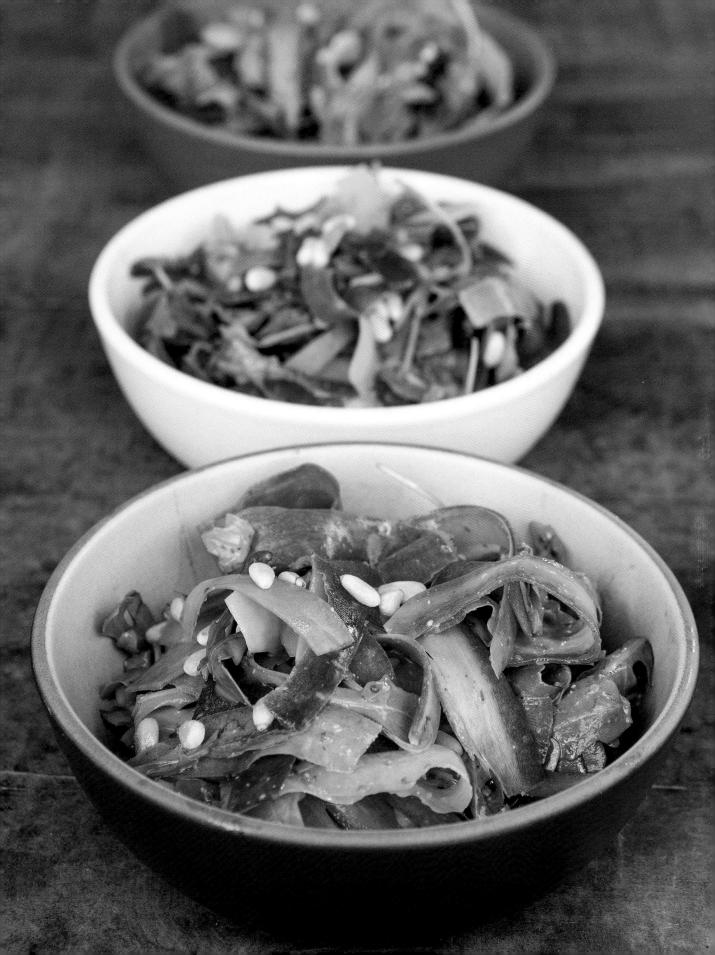

SHAVED BRUSSELS SPROUT–APPLE SALAD WITH HAZELNUTS

Brussels sprouts are high in sulfur, glucosinolate, and vitamin C, making them a great detox food. Shredding them into small pieces means they are easily palatable, and with the sweetness of the apple and classic honey-lemon dressing, you'll find yourself craving this salad often.

MAKES 4 SERVINGS
PREP TIME: 30 MINUTES

SALAD

5 cups (440 g) finely shredded brussels sprouts (about 16 sprouts)

1 red apple, thinly sliced

⅓ cup (38 g) raw hazelnuts, chopped

DRESSING

¼ cup (60 ml) olive oil

2 tablespoons (28 ml) lemon juice

1 teaspoon whole grain Dijon mustard

1 teaspoon raw honey

Salt to taste

FOR THE SALAD

Use a mandoline or a knife to finely shred the brussels sprouts and slice the apple. Toss together with the hazelnuts in a large bowl.

FOR THE DRESSING

Whisk or briefly pulse the ingredients in a mini blender and toss with the salad.

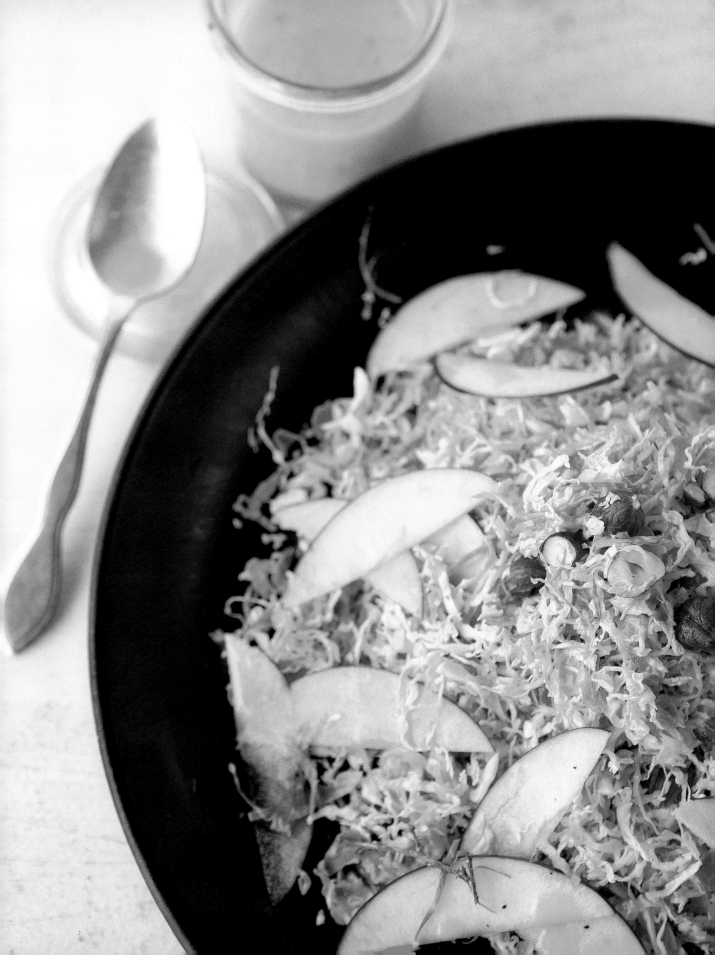

DANDELION-FENNEL SALAD

Dandelion greens make a great detox salad. They purify the blood, detoxify the liver, boost the immune system, help heal skin conditions, and support kidney and brain function. They're rich in vitamin K, calcium, and iron, as well as many other vitamins and minerals. Their bitterness is balanced by the dates, while the fennel and grapefruit add a fragrant freshness.

MAKES 2 SERVINGS
PREP TIME: 15 MINUTES

1 bunch of dandelion greens, chopped

1 large bulb of fennel, shaved or finely chopped

1 grapefruit, supremed

3 to 4 Medjool dates, pitted and diced

3 tablespoons (45 ml) lemon juice

3 tablespoons (45 ml) olive oil

Salt and pepper to taste

Toss all the ingredients in a large bowl and serve.

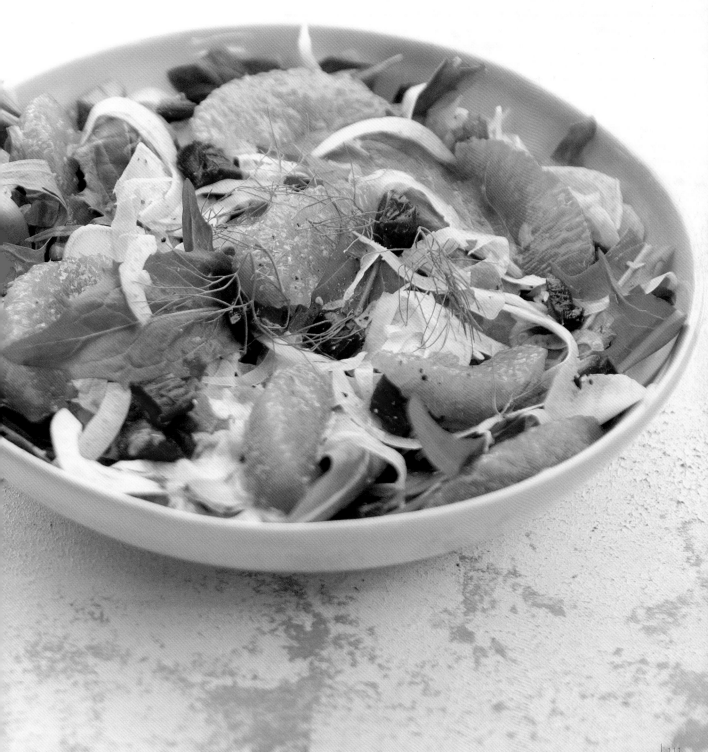

CHINESE CABBAGE SALAD WITH ORANGE TAHINI DRESSING

Fragrant, sweet, and tart orange is the star of this colorful, crunchy salad. If you have leftovers, it makes a great breakfast the following day. Just don't toss with the dressing until you're ready to eat.

MAKES 2 TO 4 SERVINGS
PREP TIME: 30 MINUTES
PLAN AHEAD: SOAK ¼ CUP (36 G) RAW ALMONDS FOR 8 TO 12 HOURS OR OVERNIGHT AND RINSE WELL. PINCH OFF THE SKINS, IF YOU LIKE, AND CHOP.

DRESSING

½ cup (120 g) raw tahini

½ cup (120 ml) freshly squeezed orange juice

3 tablespoons (45 ml) coconut aminos

2 tablespoons (28 ml) Bragg apple cider vinegar

2 teaspoons raw honey or 1 tablespoon (14 g) coconut nectar

1 teaspoon orange zest

1 small clove of garlic

Dash of cayenne pepper

SALAD

2 cups (140 g) shredded Napa cabbage

2 cups (140 g) shredded purple cabbage

⅓ cup (5 g) chopped cilantro

⅓ cup (33 g) sliced green onions

2 radishes, thinly sliced with a mandoline

2 to 3 oranges, supremed

¼ cup (36 g) raw almonds, soaked 8 to 12 hours, rinsed, and chopped

FOR THE DRESSING
Blend all the ingredients until smooth.

FOR THE SALAD
Toss all the ingredients in a large bowl and drizzle with the dressing.

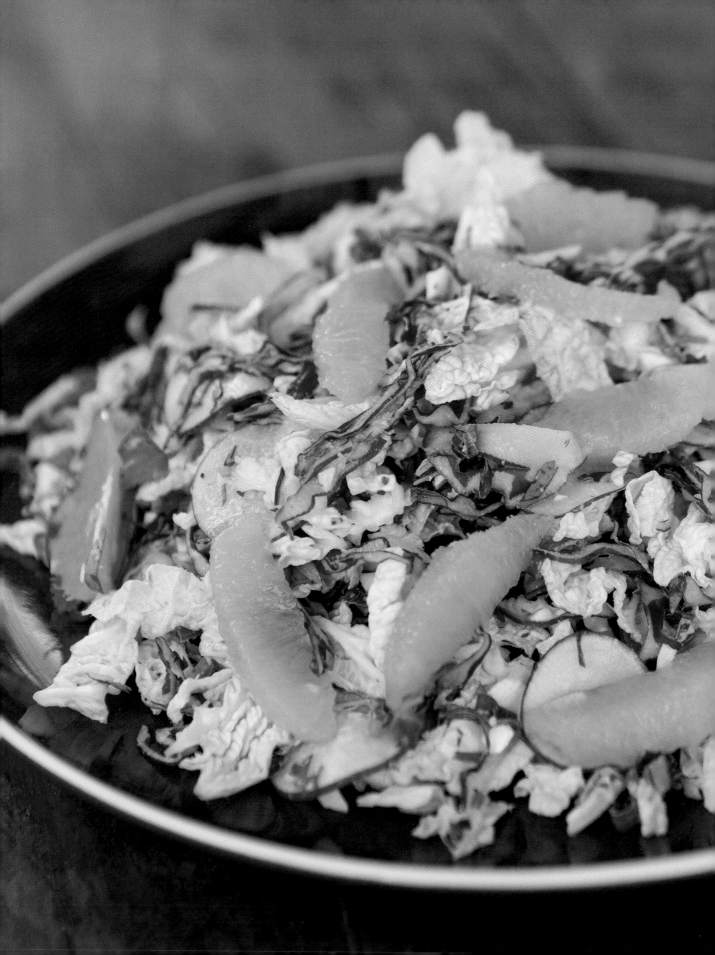

KALE IS KIND SALAD ▶

This popular apple, walnut, and date salad combo is often served with salty pancetta. I substituted black Botija olives instead. If you can't find them at your local grocery, you can use any salted olive you like.

MAKES 2 TO 3 SERVINGS
PREP TIME: 20 MINUTES
PLAN AHEAD: SOAK ¼ CUP (25 G) RAW WALNUTS FOR 4 TO 6 HOURS, RINSE, AND DRAIN.

1 bunch of kale, destemmed and chopped

2 tablespoons (28 ml) lemon juice

¼ teaspoon sea salt

1 avocado, halved

1 apple, diced

¼ cup (25 g) raw walnuts, soaked and chopped

2 Medjool dates, pitted and chopped

¼ cup (25 g) Botija or other salty olives, chopped

Massage the chopped kale with the lemon juice and sea salt until it becomes soft and wilted. Take half of the avocado and massage it into the kale until creamy. Cube the remaining half of the avocado and toss with the kale, apples, walnuts, dates, and olives.

CUCUMBER-APPLE SALAD

Mint, yogurt, and honey go so lovely together in this crunchy medley of Middle Eastern flavors. This refreshing salad has three ingredients from my top favorite detox foods list and makes a tasty breakfast salad or a good option whenever you're in the mood for something light.

MAKES 2 SERVINGS
PREP TIME: 10 MINUTES
PLAN AHEAD: YOU WILL NEED ⅓ CUP (77 G) OF COCONUT YOGURT (PAGE 168).

1 medium cucumber, peeled and diced small

1 large granny smith apple, diced small

⅓ cup (77 g) Coconut Yogurt (page 168)

2 tablespoons (12 g) finely chopped fresh mint

1 teaspoon raw honey or to taste

Mix all the ingredients in a bowl and serve.

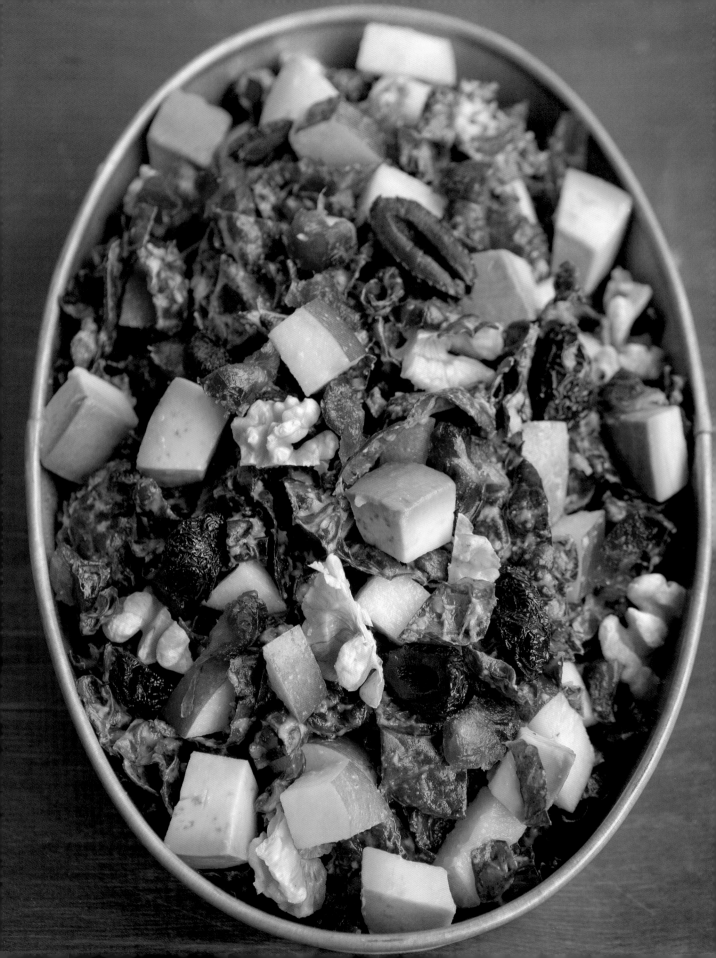

MIDDLE EASTERN BEET SALAD ▶

Tossing shredded beets with lemon, herbs, and seasonings makes them not only palatable, but addicting. I find one bowl of this salad is never enough.

MAKES 2 TO 3 SERVINGS
PREP TIME: 20 MINUTES

1 large beet, peeled and shredded

1 large carrot, peeled and shredded

¼ cup (15 g) chopped parsley

¼ cup (24 g) chopped mint

¼ cup (60 ml) lemon juice

2 tablespoons (28 ml) olive oil

1 clove of garlic, crushed

¼ teaspoon sea salt

Dash of fresh cracked pepper

(Optional) Dash of cayenne pepper

Toss all the ingredients in a medium-size bowl and serve. This is a good salad to make ahead and will last 2 days in the refrigerator.

CARROT COLESLAW

Colorful, zesty, and crunchy—this is my salad trifecta! It's a good salad to double up on since it's hearty and will last a couple of days in the fridge.

MAKES 2 SERVINGS
PREP TIME: 25 MINUTES
PLAN AHEAD: SOAK ⅓ CUP (33 G) RAW WALNUTS FOR 4 TO 6 HOURS, RINSE, AND DRAIN.

SALAD

2 cups (140 g) shredded purple cabbage

2 cups (220 g) shredded carrots

⅓ cup (33 g) coarsely chopped raw walnuts, soaked

¼ cup (4 g) chopped cilantro

DRESSING

¼ cup (60 ml) olive oil

2 tablespoons (28 ml) Bragg apple cider vinegar

1 tablespoon (14 g) coconut nectar or honey

1 small clove of garlic, crushed

Pinch of sea salt

Dash of pepper

FOR THE SALAD

Toss all the salad ingredients in a medium-size bowl.

FOR THE DRESSING

Whisk or blend all the ingredients together. Pour over the salad, toss well, and serve.

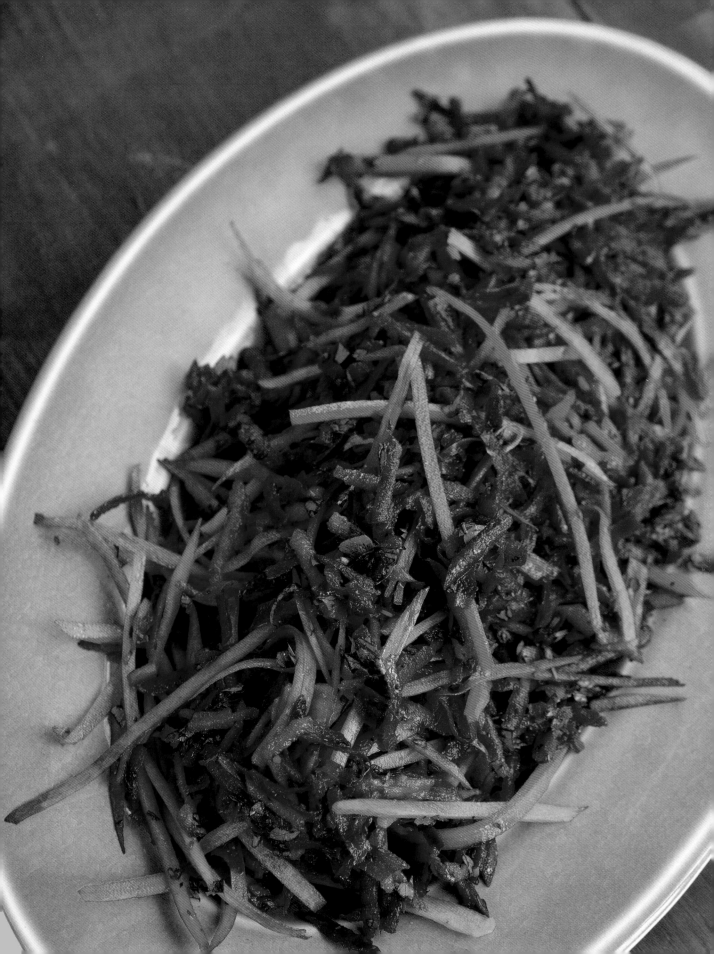

GREEK SALAD ▶

This classic Greek salad with Cashew Feta Cheese is one of my favorites and something I can always make a big bowl of to bring to friend and family dinners.

MAKES 2 SERVINGS
PREP TIME: 15 MINUTES
PLAN AHEAD: (OPTIONAL) MAKE ONE BATCH OF CASHEW FETA CHEESE (BELOW).

3 cups (141 g) chopped Romaine lettuce

1 cup (135 g) chopped cucumber

1 large tomato

¼ cup (25 g) Botija or kalamata olives

¼ of a small red onion, sliced thinly

2 tablespoons (28 ml) olive oil

2 tablespoons (28 ml) lemon juice

¼ cup (24 g) chopped mint

1 clove of garlic, crushed

⅛ teaspoon dried oregano

Salt and pepper to taste

(Optional) Cashew Feta Cheese (below), to taste.

Toss all ingredients in a large bowl until well combined.

CASHEW FETA CHEESE

Use this cheese in the Greek Salad or in any salad that needs a little flair. You can also use it as a spread on raw crackers or wraps.

MAKES 1 CUP
PREP TIME: 5 MINUTES
PLAN AHEAD: SOAK 1 CUP OF CASHEWS FOR 2 HOURS.

1 cup (140 g) cashews, soaked 2 hours

2 tablespoons (28 ml) olive oil

2 tablespoons (28 ml) lemon juice

⅛ teaspoon sea salt

Pulse all of the ingredients in a food processor, scraping down sides of container as needed until you achieve a feta consistency.

CHEF TIP: To make it even cheesier, add a little nutritional yeast before blending.

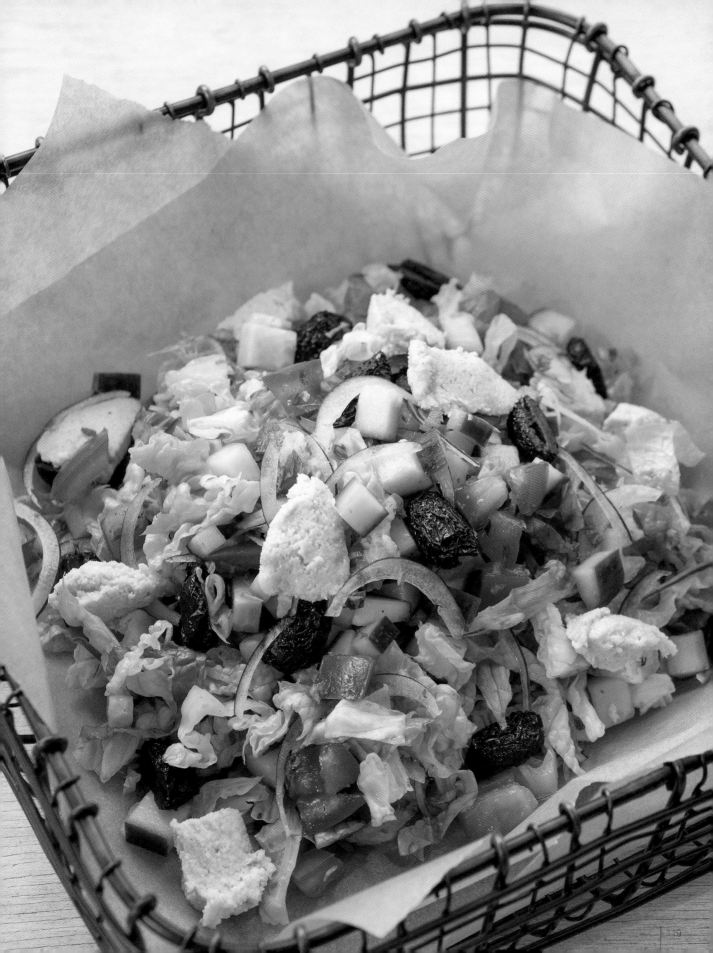

ASIAN BOK CHOY SALAD

I use a mild-tasting seaweed called dulse in this salad. It requires no soaking and can be eaten straight out of the bag. It's mineral-rich and high in thyroid-supporting iodine, B$_6$, potassium, and iron. I like to call it seaweed for people who hate seaweed, but if you're really not a fan, go ahead and omit it.

MAKES 4 SERVINGS
PREP TIME: 25 MINUTES

DRESSING

⅓ cup (80 ml) lemon juice

2 tablespoons (28 g) coconut nectar or sweetener of choice

1½ tablespoons (23 ml) olive oil

1 tablespoon (15 g) coconut aminos

2 teaspoons fresh grated ginger

¼ teaspoon crushed red pepper flakes

SALAD

4 to 6 bunches of baby bok choy, green and white portions chopped

8 skinny asparagus stalks, sliced on a bias

4 radishes, thinly sliced

1½ cups (105 g) shredded red cabbage

½ cup (40 g) dulse pieces (optional)

1 tablespoon (8 g) black sesame seeds

FOR THE DRESSING
Whisk all the ingredients in a small bowl.

FOR THE SALAD
Toss all ingredients in a large bowl and serve with the dressing.

HEALTH NOTE:
Bok choy is a card-carrying member of the anticancer cruciferous family. It's a great source of calcium; iron; vitamins A, C, and K; potassium; and folate. Baby bok choy is sweeter and milder than its grown-up version, but both are very pleasant in salads and juices. It's a great green to make a regular staple in any healthy kitchen.

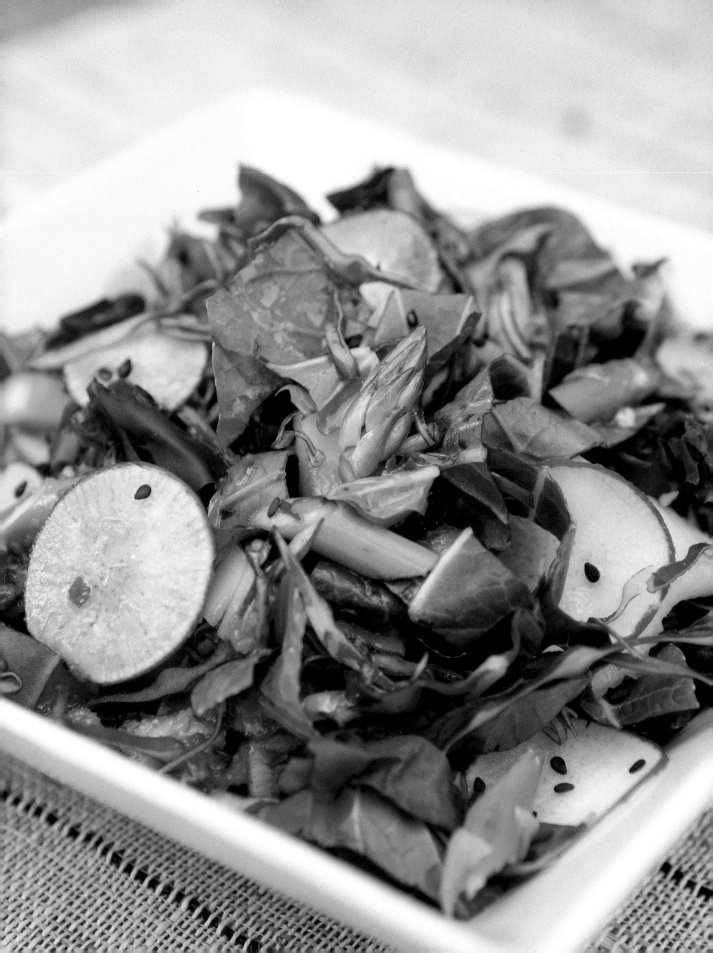

GRAPEFRUIT-AVOCADO SALAD ▶

This salad tastes fresh and light, but it is actually quite filling. If you use sweeter grapefruits, I suggest dressing the salad with lemon juice; if you have very tart grapefruits, use orange juice to balance the flavors.

MAKES 1 TO 2 SERVINGS
PREP TIME: 25 MINUTES

Half a bunch kale, stems removed and leaves finely chopped

2 grapefruits, supremed

1 avocado, cubed

¼ cup (24 g) chopped mint

2 tablespoons (28 ml) lemon or orange juice

1½ tablespoons (30 g) raw honey

Toss all the ingredients in a medium-size bowl and serve.

THE QUICKIE SALAD

When I only have a few minutes to throw something together, this is my go-to salad. Don't be fooled by its simplicity—it can really hit the spot. Feel free to jazz it up with a few olives, cubed avocado, or a dollop of Beanless Spinach Hummus (page 165).

MAKES 1 SERVING
PREP TIME: 5 MINUTES

1 head of Romaine or other lettuce, or half of prepackaged mixed greens

2 tablespoons (28 ml) olive oil

2 tablespoons (28 ml) lemon juice

1 small clove of garlic, crushed

Small handful of dulse strips

Dash of spirulina

Salt and pepper to taste

Place all the ingredients in a large bowl and toss until well combined.

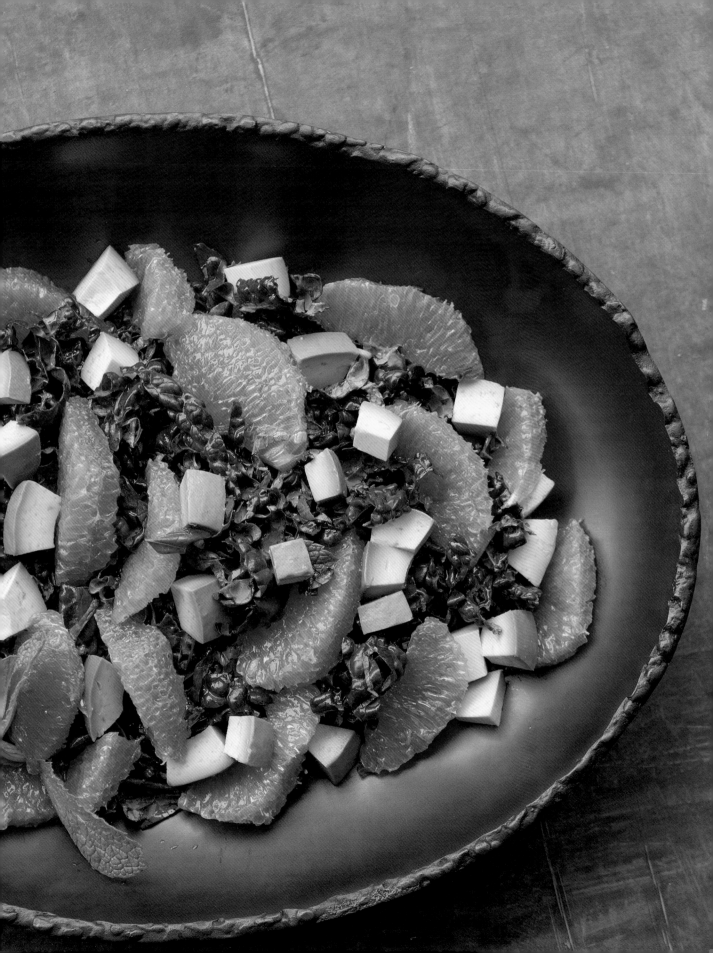

ROASTED BEETS (COOKED)

Beets are a fantastic detox food. I enjoy them year round, but when it's cooler, I prefer to roast them. Toss cooked beets into salads or try them in the Zesty Beet Salad recipe below or Dilly Beet Soup on page 98.

MAKES 3 CUPS (408 G)
PREP TIME: ABOUT 1 HOUR PLUS TIME TO COOL

2 medium-size beets

Preheat oven to 400°F (200°C, or gas mark 6). Wash and trim the beets. Dry them very well and then wrap individually in foil.

Place on a baking sheet or pan and bake for about 45 to 60 minutes, depending on the size. Poke the beets with a fork to check for doneness; they're ready when you can easily pierce them.

Allow the beets to cool and then use your fingers to slip the skin off. Gloves are highly recommended if you don't want to look like you just murdered someone.

Chop the beets and store them in a glass container for up to one week.

ZESTY BEET SALAD (COOKED) ▶

MAKES 1 SERVING
PREP TIME: 10 MINUTES

2 medium-size roasted beets, diced (about 3 cups or 408 g)

2 tablespoons (8 g) chopped dill

2 tablespoons (28 ml) lemon juice

1 tablespoon (15 ml) olive oil

Salt and pepper to taste

Toss all the ingredients in a medium-size bowl and serve.

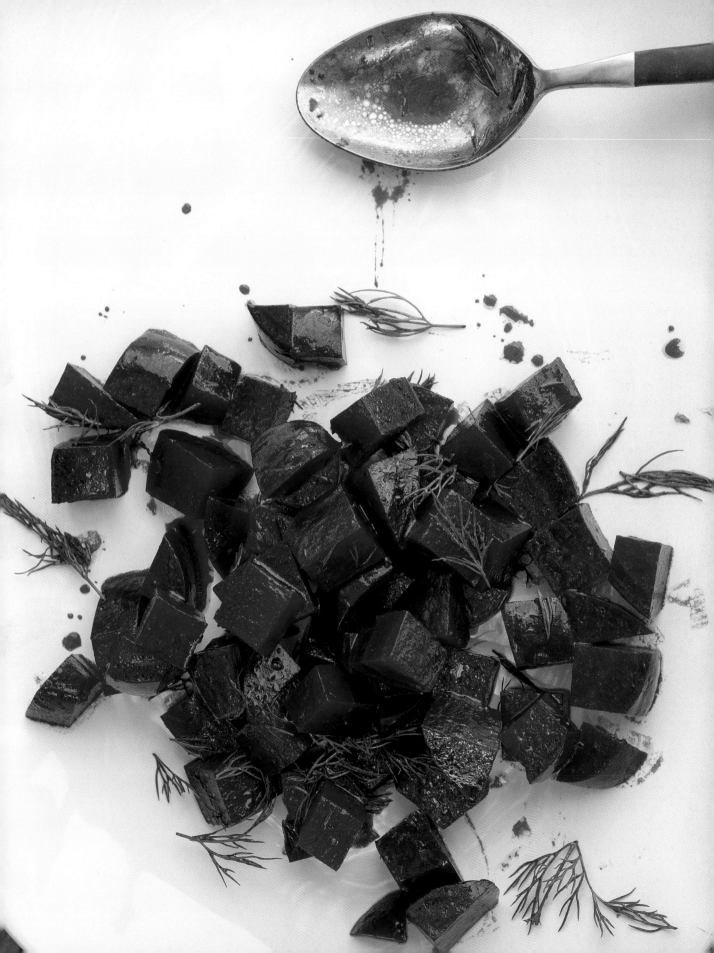

SALAD DRESSINGS

CLASSIC CAESAR

MAKES 1 CUP (235 ML)

¾ cup (175 ml) olive oil

¼ cup (60 ml) lemon juice

1 tablespoon (16 g) chickpea miso paste

1 tablespoon (15 g) raw tahini

1 tablespoon (9 g) capers

2 teaspoons Dijon mustard

1 clove of garlic

Fresh cracked pepper to taste

Process all the ingredients in a blender on low speed until smooth.

ORANGE TAHINI DRESSING

MAKES 1 CUP (235 ML)

½ cup (120 g) raw tahini

½ cup (120 ml) orange juice

3 tablespoons (45 g) coconut aminos

2 tablespoons (28 ml) Bragg apple cider vinegar

2 teaspoons raw honey or 1 tablespoon (14 g) coconut nectar

1 teaspoon orange zest

1 small clove of garlic

Dash of cayenne

Process all the ingredients in a blender until smooth.

FRESH HERB AND LEMON DRESSING

MAKES 1½ CUPS (355 ML)

⅔ cup (160 ml) olive oil

½ cup (120 ml) lemon juice

¼ cup (12 g) fresh, finely chopped chives

¼ cup (10 g) fresh, finely chopped basil

1½ tablespoons (30 g) raw honey or coconut nectar

1 tablespoon (15 g) whole grain Dijon mustard

Sea salt and ground pepper to taste

Pulse all the ingredients in a blender until combined. Do not overblend.

GARLIC TAHINI DRESSING
MAKES ABOUT 1 CUP (235 ML)

½ cup (120 g) raw tahini

⅓ cup (80 ml) water

¼ cup (60 ml) lemon juice

2 cloves of garlic

¼ teaspoon sea salt

⅛ teaspoon black pepper

Place all the ingredients into a blender and blend until smooth. This dressing will thicken during storage. Add 1 tablespoon (15 ml) of water at a time to thin.

HEMP SEED RANCH DRESSING
MAKES 1 CUP (235 ML)

1 cup (120 g) hemp seeds

½ cup (120 ml) water

⅓ cup (80 ml) lemon juice

1 tablespoon (16 g) chickpea miso paste

1 clove of garlic

¼ teaspoon sea salt

1 tablespoon (4 g) chopped dill

1 tablespoon (4 g) chopped parsely

Dash of fresh pepper

Blend all the ingredients until smooth. Adjust seasonings to taste. You can use other herbs such as chives, tarragon, or sage.

SWEET BASIL DRESSING
MAKES 1 CUP (235 ML)

1 cup (40 g) loosely packed fresh basil

½ cup (67.5 g) raw cashews, soaked 2 hours

⅓ cup (80 ml) water

¼ cup (60 ml) lemon juice

1½ tablespoons (21 g) coconut nectar

1 tablespoon (16 g) chickpea miso paste

1 teaspoon coconut aminos

1 clove of garlic

Process all the ingredients in a blender until smooth.

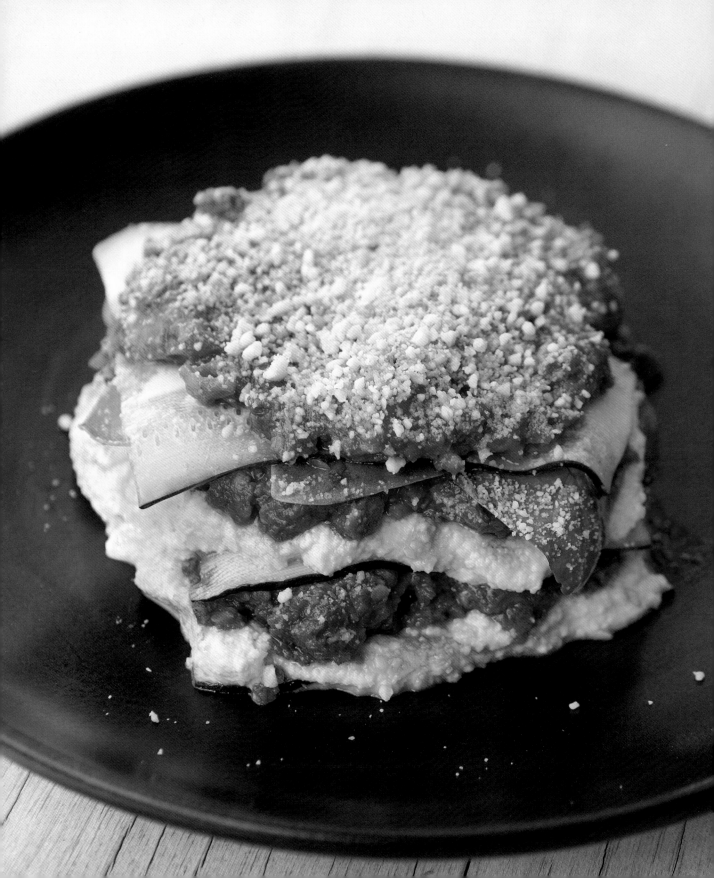

RUSTIC RAW LASAGNA

This recipe takes a little extra effort, but you will have enough left over to have it again the next day. It's well worth it if you have a hankering for Italian.

MAKES 2 SERVINGS
PREP TIME: 35 MINUTES
PLAN AHEAD: SOAK THE FOLLOWING INGREDIENTS:

- ⅓ cup (33 g) raw walnuts for four to six hours
- ½ cup (28 g) sun-dried tomatoes in hot water for 1 to 2 hours
- ¼ cup (35 g) raw pine nuts for 2 hours
- ¼ cup (35 g) raw cashews for 2 hours

(Optional) Make Parmesan "Cheese" (page 167).

LASAGNA

1 medium-size zucchini

1 cup (30 g) baby spinach, packed

2 tablespoons (28 ml) olive oil

⅛ teaspoon sea salt

RICOTTA

⅓ cup (45 g) raw pine nuts, soaked

⅓ cup (47 g) raw cashews, soaked

2 tablespoons (28 ml) water

1½ tablespoons (5 g) nutritional yeast

2 teaspoons lemon juice

¼ teaspoon sea salt

BOLOGNESE SAUCE

½ cup (28 g) soaked sun-dried tomatoes, drained well

⅓ cup (33 g) soaked raw walnuts

Few leaves of fresh basil, chopped, or ¼ teaspoon dried basil

½ teaspoon dried Italian seasoning

1 small Medjool date, pitted

1 clove of garlic, crushed

Dash of crushed red pepper

¼ teaspoon sea salt

FOR THE LASAGNA

Slice the zucchini lengthwise into six thin planks using a mandoline or a knife. Then cut each plank in half so you have twelve rectangular pieces (six pieces for each lasagna serving).

In a medium-size bowl, toss the spinach, olive oil, and sea salt and give everything a light massage. Allow the mixture to marinate while you make the sauce and cheese.

NOTE: If you have thick zucchini planks, add them to the mixture as well to soften.

FOR THE RICOTTA

Process all ingredients in a food processor until smooth. Scrape down the sides as needed until well blended.

FOR THE SAUCE

Process all the ingredients in a food processor, scraping down sides as needed. I like to leave it slightly chunky.

TO ASSEMBLE

Lay down two pieces of zucchini on a plate, side by side, and top with a thin layer of ricotta followed by a generous layer of Bolognese sauce. Top with spinach and repeat the layers again. Top with additional sauce, a light drizzle of olive oil, and a sprinkle of Parmesan "Cheese" (page 167).

STRAWBERRY CHIA PARFAIT

Chia pudding is a staple in my kitchen. I've made it a million different ways, but this is how I enjoy it best. Just berries, walnuts, and some cinnamon make this an ultra simple but super satisfying breakfast or dessert. Kick it up a notch with a sprinkle of cacao nibs.

MAKES 2 SERVINGS
PREP TIME: 15 MINUTES PLUS 6 HOURS OR OVERNIGHT
PLAN AHEAD: MAKE ALMOND MILK (PAGE 70) OR COCONUT MILK (PAGE 72).

2 cups (475 ml) Almond Milk (page 70) or Coconut Milk (page 72)

⅓ cup (69 g) chia seeds

2 tablespoons (28 ml) xylitol granules, a few drops of liquid stevia, or your favorite sweetener, to taste

2 cups fresh or frozen (290 g or 510 g) strawberries, thawed if necessary

¼ cup (30 g) chopped raw walnuts

Dash of cinnamon

Mix the almond or coconut milk with the chia seeds. Let it sit for five minutes and then mix again, removing any clumps. Soak for 6 hours or overnight in the refrigerator. Sweeten to taste.

Mash the strawberries with a fork or pulse very briefly in a food processor, keeping the chunky consistency. Sweeten to taste if desired.

To serve, alternate layering the chia pudding and strawberries in a small mason jar or glass and top with chopped walnuts and a dash of cinnamon.

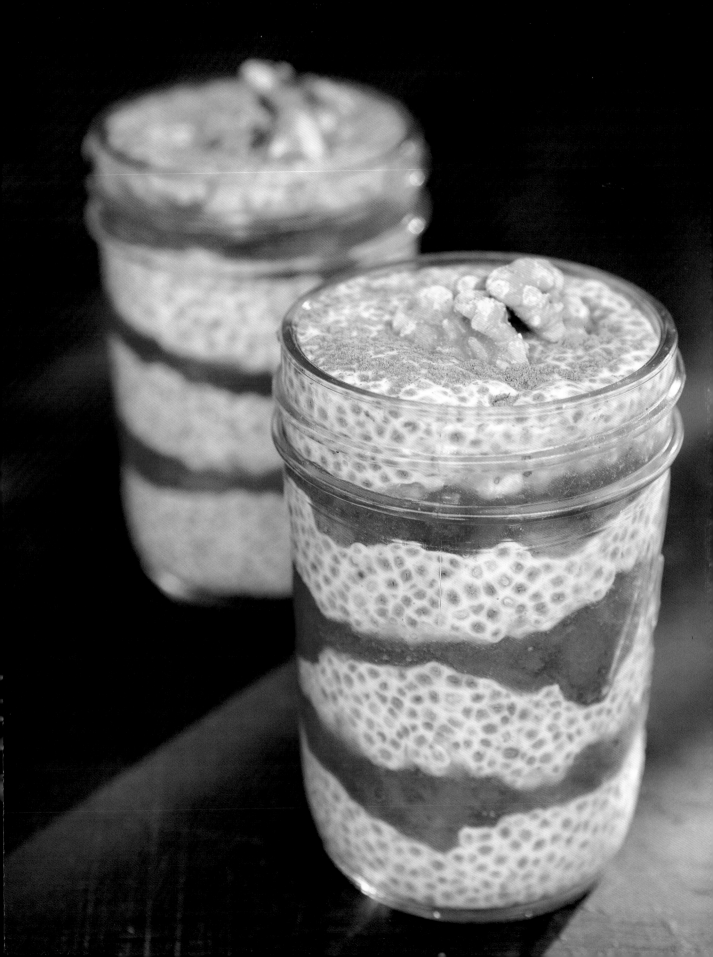

HONEY-BERRY COCONUT ▶ YOGURT BREAKFAST

This one is for those of you who need an uber-quick and portable breakfast.

MAKES 1 TO 2 SERVINGS
PREP TIME: 5 MINUTES
PLAN AHEAD: YOU WILL NEED ½ CUP (115 G) COCONUT YOGURT (PAGE 168) AND 2 TABLESPOONS (28 G) OF YOUR FAVORITE RAW NUTS, SOAKED. MY FAVORITE NUTS TO USE ARE ALMONDS, WALNUTS, AND PECANS.

1 cup (145 g) of your favorite fresh berries

½ cup (115 g) Coconut Yogurt (page 168)

2 tablespoons (28 g) soaked and chopped raw almonds, walnuts, or pecans

1 tablespoon (20 g) raw honey

Place the berries in a small mason jar or bowl (or coconut) and top with the yogurt, nuts, and honey.

BERRY MUESLI CEREAL

Use your favorite berries in this European-inspired muesli, as well as any other modifications like adding pecans, walnuts, hemp seeds, dried fruit, cinnamon, cardamom, mesquite, or whatever floats your boat.

MAKES 1 SERVINGS
PREP TIME: 10 MINUTES
PLAN AHEAD: SOAK 1 TO 2 TABLESPOONS (9 TO 18 G) RAW ALMONDS FOR 8 TO 12 HOURS THE NIGHT BEFORE AND THEN DRAIN AND RINSE. PINCH THE ALMONDS TO REMOVE THE SKINS. YOU'LL ALSO WANT TO HAVE SOME ALMOND MILK (PAGE 70) ON HAND.

1 to 2 tablespoons (9 to 18 g) raw almonds, soaked overnight, rinsed and chopped

2 tablespoons (10 g) shredded coconut

1 tablespoon (13 g) chia seeds

½ tablespoon ground flax seed

1 tablespoon (6 g) goji berries or raisins

Dash of vanilla powder or ½ teaspoon vanilla extract

Combine all the ingredients in a bowl and top with the almond milk. Allow it to sit for five minutes. Sweeten to taste with your favorite sweetener.

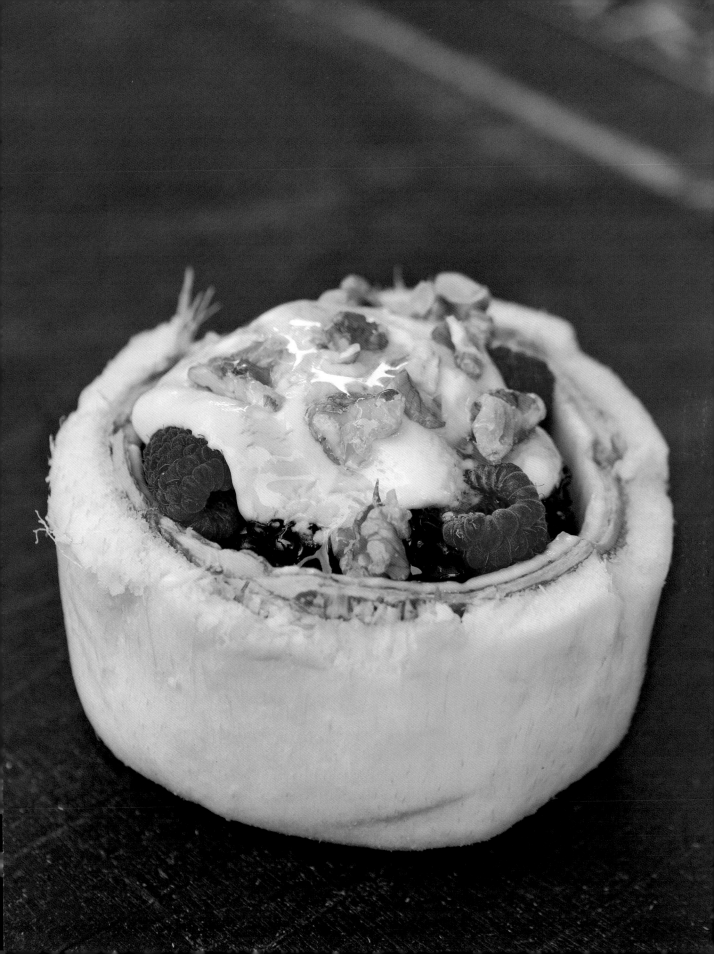

ROMAINE FRESCO TACOS

The fresh flavors and crunchy texture of these tacos make me feel like I should be dining al fresco on a beach in Tulum. I crave these on a regular basis and enjoy them rolled up in lettuce leaves as much as just eating it straight out of the bowl. For the best results, keep your dices small.

MAKES 2 TO 3 SERVINGS
PREP TIME: 30 MINUTES

2 Roma tomatoes, diced

1 mango, diced

1 small avocado, diced

½ cup (70 g) diced cucumber

½ cup (65 g) diced jicama

1 jalapeño, seeded and diced

2 tablespoons (20 g) diced red onion

2 tablespoons (2 g) chopped cilantro

2 tablespoons (15 g) hemp seeds

1 tablespoon (15 ml) lime juice

Dash of cayenne pepper

Sea salt, to taste

2 to 3 leaves Romaine letuce or cabbage

Mix all the ingredients together and spoon onto the Romaine lettuce or cabbage leaves.

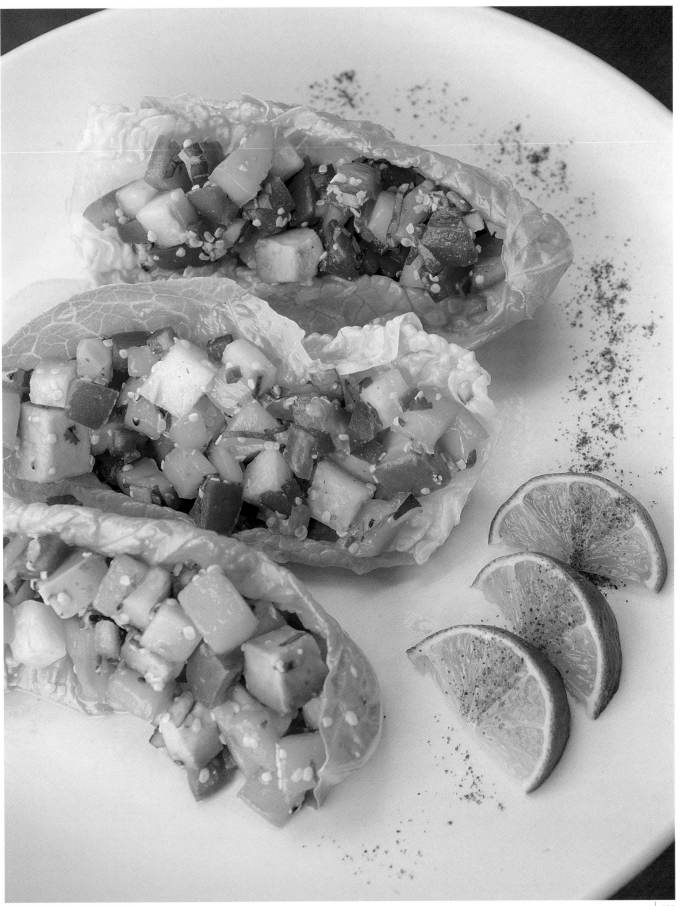

135

GINGER-MISO VEGGIE ROLLS

The great thing about these rolls is that you can customize them so many different ways or just use up what you have in the fridge. The ginger-miso spread is packed with flavor and complements any combination you come up with. What's my favorite combo? Avocado, cucumber, carrots, Quick Pickled Cabbage (page 169), and broccoli sprouts.

MAKES 4 TO 6 ROLLS
PREP TIME: 30 MINUTES
PLAN AHEAD: SOAK 1 CUP (145 G) SUNFLOWER SEEDS FOR 4 TO 6 HOURS,

GINGER-MISO SPREAD

1 cup (145 g) sunflower seeds, soaked 4 to 6 hours, drained, and rinsed

¼ cup (63 g) chickpea miso paste

1 tablespoon (15 ml) Bragg apple cider vinegar

1 tablespoon (8 g) grated ginger

1 tablespoon (14 g) coconut nectar

1 clove of garlic, crushed

FOR THE ROLLS

1 package of raw or toasted nori sheets

FILLING OPTIONS

Avocado

Cucumber

Carrot

Sprouts

Mango

Asparagus

Zucchini

Bell pepper

Romaine lettuce

Grated beet

Quick Pickled Cabbage (page 169)

FOR THE SPREAD

Process all the ingredients in a food processor until it becomes a paste. Scrape down the sides of the container as needed.

TO ASSEMBLE

Place one nori sheet, shiny side down, on a sushi mat or cutting board. Slather the ginger-miso spread over bottom third of sheet and top with the filling options. (Don't overdo it!) Roll from the bottom up until about 1 inch (2.5 cm) of nori is showing. Dab some water on the edge of the nori sheet and finish rolling. This will seal the roll.

Use a very sharp knife to cut your rolls into the desired-size pieces.

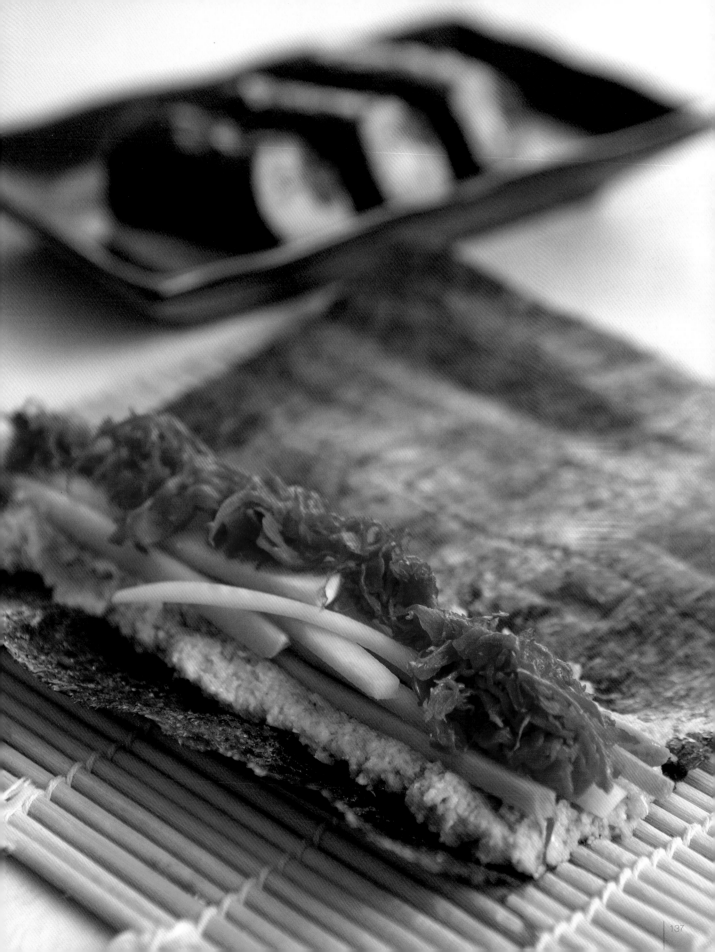

GREEN SUBMARINE WRAP

Collard greens make awesome raw wraps. They hold up well and are hearty as well as nutritious. Look for the largest collard leaves when picking them out of the store. You can customize the filling to whatever floats your boat. Below is my favorite combo, but the possibilities are endless.

MAKES 2 TO 4 SERVINGS
PREP TIME: 15 MINUTES
PLAN AHEAD: MAKE ONE BATCH OF BEANLESS SPINACH HUMMUS (PAGE 165) OR POWER PESTO SPREAD (PAGE 166) AND QUICK PICKLED CABBAGE (PAGE 169).

FOR THE WRAPS

2 to 4 collard leaves

FOR THE FILLING

Beanless Spinach Hummus (page 165) or Power Pesto Spread (page 166)

Quick Pickled Cabbage (page 169)

Tomato, seeded and sliced

Avocado, sliced

Red onion, thinly sliced

Broccoli sprouts

Botija olives

OTHER FILLING OPTIONS

Romaine lettuce

Bell pepper strips

Julienned carrots

Cucumber sticks

Asparagus spears

Sunflower sprouts or your favorite sprouts

Fresh herbs like mint, basil, or chives

Dulse strips

Tahini Dressing (page 142)

Ginger-Miso spread (page 136)

Queen of Green Dip (page 169)

TO PREPARE THE COLLARD LEAVES

Cut off the part of the stem that comes out from the leaf and fillet the main stem with a paring knife to make it more flexible.

TO ASSEMBLE

Spread the desired amount of hummus or pesto over the bottom half of a collard leaf. Layer with the desired ingredients and then roll from the bottom up, tucking the sides in as you go along to make a nice, tight wrap.

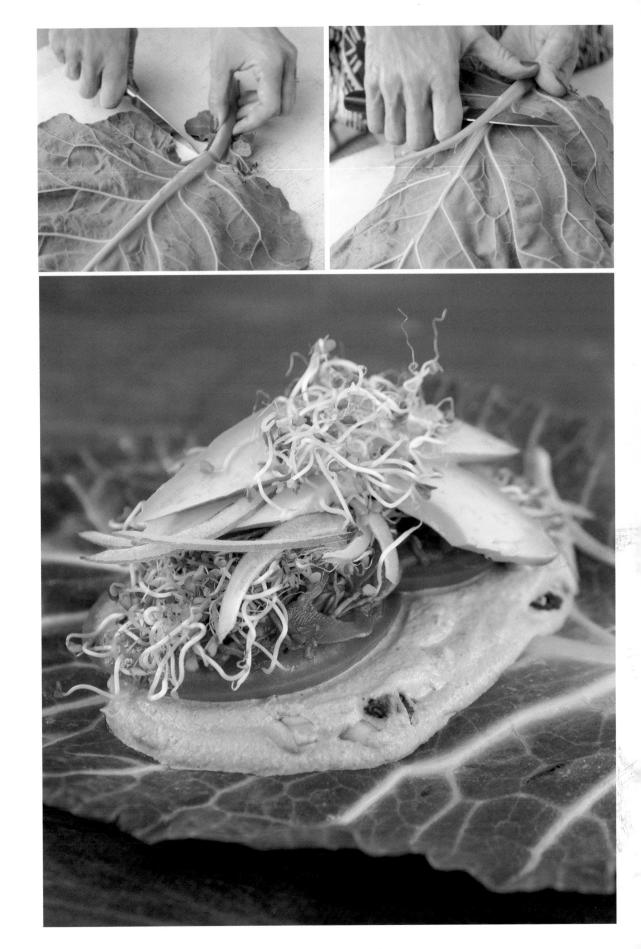

ZUCCHINI NOODLES AL DENTE

Zucchini noodles are a favorite in the raw food world. The taste is neutral, especially if you decide to peel them, and they take on the flavor of whatever sauce you dress them in. They shine best in Italian flavors. Below is my light and lovely noodle recipe that can all be tossed easily in one bowl. I also included a couple of my classic raw Italian sauces on pages 166 and 167 if you want something more familiar. They work great slightly warmed, too! And they're even better topped with a little Parmesan "Cheese" (page 167).

To prepare the zucchini noodles, use a vegetable spiralizer (I really like the one from World Cuisine) or use a hand peeler to turn them into linguini-style ribbons.

MAKES 2 SERVINGS
PREP TIME: 15 MINUTES

2 zucchini, spiralized or peeled into ribbons

2 Roma tomatoes, diced

½ of a small bell pepper, diced

¼ cup (25 g) chopped Botija olives

¼ cup (35 g) raw pine nuts

1 to 2 tablespoons (15 to 28 ml) olive oil

1 tablespoon (3 g) chopped fresh basil

1 small clove of garlic, crushed

Salt and pepper, to taste

Light squeeze of fresh lemon juice

Toss all the ingredients in a bowl and serve.

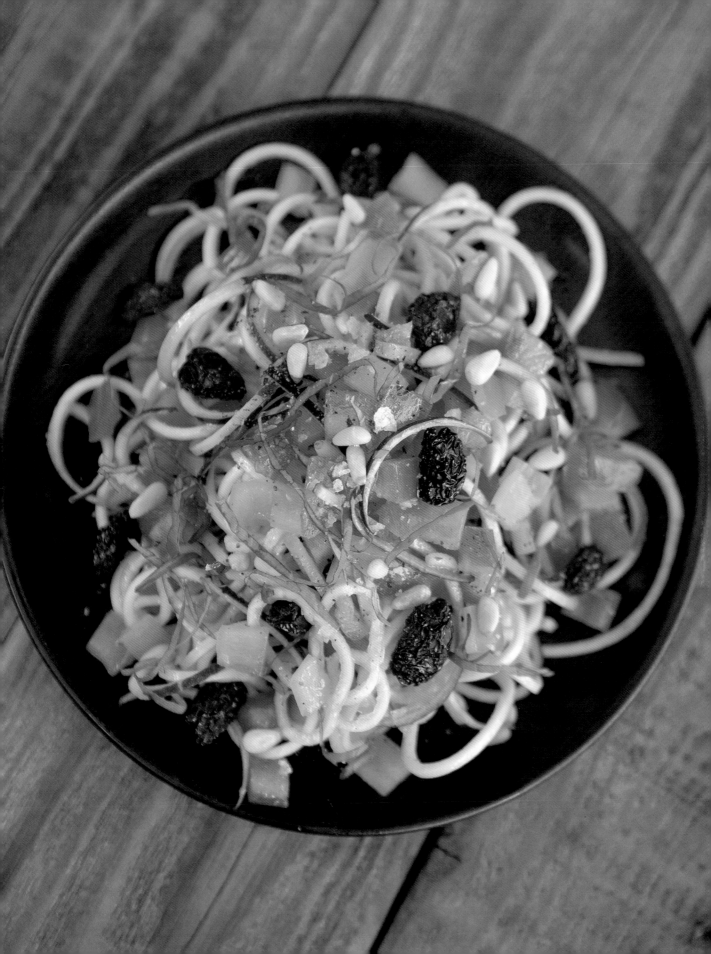

TABBOULEH SALAD WRAP

It's amazing that something that tastes so good is also doing so much good for our body. Cauliflower contains anticancer compounds while helping to remove excess estrogen. Parsley is anti-inflammatory, tomatoes are high in antioxidants, mint is a digestive aid, garlic is great for the immune system, and lemon is our favorite liver and gallbladder cleanser.

MAKES 2 TO 4 SERVINGS
PREP TIME: 30 MINUTES

TAHINI DRESSING

½ cup (120 g) raw tahini

⅓ cup (80 ml) water

¼ cup (60 ml) lemon juice

2 cloves of garlic

¼ teaspoon sea salt

⅛ teaspoon black pepper

(Optional) Dash of cayenne pepper

TABBOULEH

2 cups (200 g) chopped cauliflower florets

1 bunch of parsley, stems removed and
    leaves chopped

¼ cup (24 g) fresh mint

1 large tomato, seeded and diced

¼ cup (30 g) hemp seeds

2 tablespoons (20 g) yellow onion, chopped

2 to 3 tablespoons (28 to 45 ml) lemon juice

2 tablespoons (30 ml) olive oil

½ teaspoon sea salt

Fresh cracked pepper to taste

4 to 6 Romaine lettuce leaves for wrap

FOR THE TAHINI DRESSING
Place all the ingredients into a blender and process until smooth. Adjust seasonings to taste.

FOR THE TABBOULEH
Pulse the cauliflower in a food processor until broken down into rice-size pieces. Transfer to a medium bowl. Add the parsley and mint to the food processor and pulse several times until finely chopped.

Transfer the herbs to the bowl with cauliflower and add the remaining ingredients. Toss well. Adjust seasonings to taste.

Serve the tabbouleh over Romaine leaves and drizzle with the tahini dressing. You can eat this as a wrap or cut up as a salad.

The tabbouleh is even tastier the next day, but it should be eaten within 2 days.

NOTE: Store leftover dressing separately for up to 5 days in the refrigerator. If it thickens, just stir in 1 tablespoon (15 ml) of water at a time to thin.

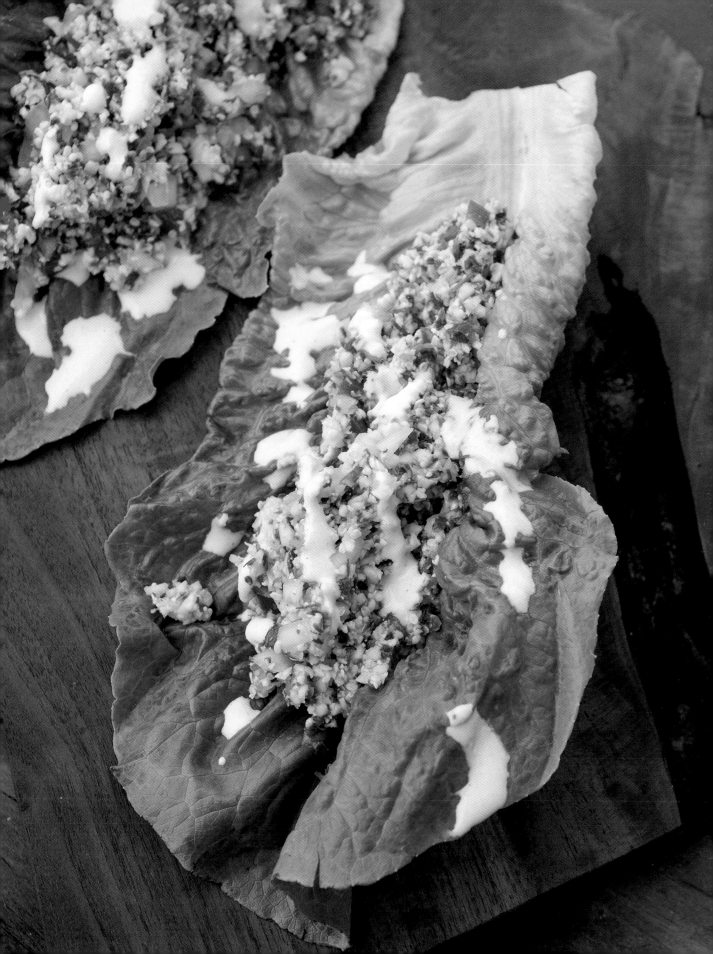

SWEET AND SPICY KELP NOODLES

Kelp noodles can be found in the refrigerated section of your health food store and are so much fun to play with in recipes. Basically, they're just a carrier for sauce because they take on the flavor of anything you dress them in. Plus, they're calorie-free and supersatisfying, especially in this ridiculously good sweet-and-spicy "peanut"-style sauce.

MAKES 2 SERVINGS
PREP TIME: 30 MINUTES

SAUCE

½ cup (130 g) raw almond butter

¼ cup (60 ml) coconut aminos

3 tablespoons (45 ml) brown rice vinegar

2 tablespoons (28 g) coconut nectar

1 tablespoon (8 g) grated ginger

2 cloves of garlic, crushed

¼ teaspoon crushed red pepper

NOODLES

1 package of kelp noodles

2 cups (134 g) finely shredded kale

½ of a red bell pepper, sliced thinly with a mandoline

2 carrots, julienned or cut into ribbons with a vegetable peeler

1 scallion, green and white parts thinly sliced

¼ cup (35 g) chopped raw cashews

FOR THE SAUCE
Blend all the ingredients until smooth.

FOR THE NOODLES
Rinse and separate the kelp noodles. Drain all the liquid very well and transfer to a large bowl. I recommend cutting the noodles with kitchen scissors to make them easier to eat.

Toss the noodles with the sauce and remaining ingredients except for the cashews.

This tastes best if warmed gently over the stovetop or in a dehydrator for 1 hour at 145°F (63°C). Divide into two bowls and sprinkle with chopped cashews.

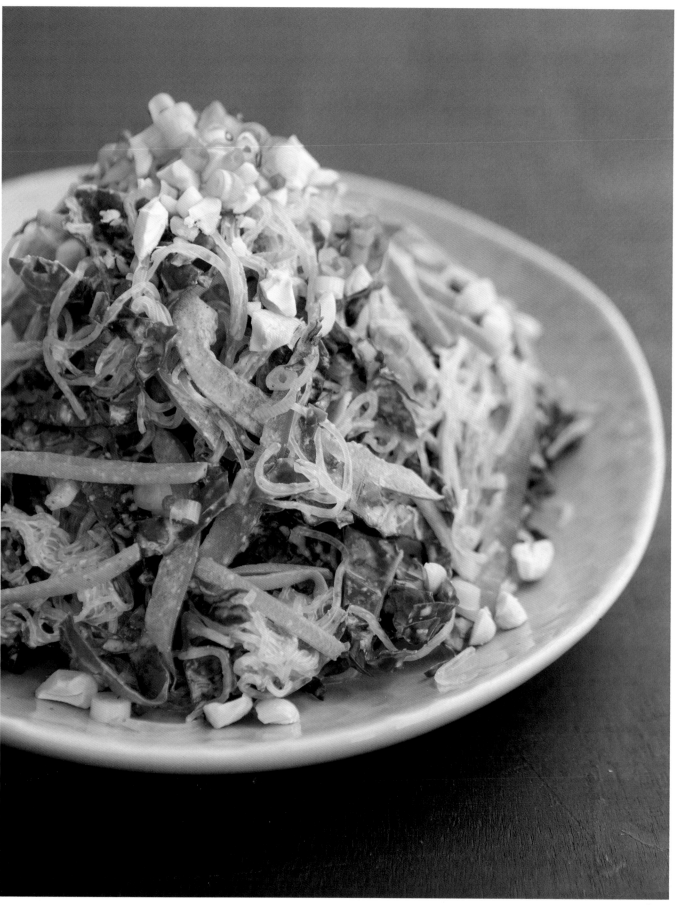

ASIAN ROOT WRAPS

This crunchy and creamy fresh wrap only involves four ingredients and reminds me of Vietnamese-style spring rolls. Use a mandoline to make thin, pliable wrappers and play around with the filling if you want. You can even throw in some small lettuce leaves for some extra green.

MAKES 2 SERVINGS
PREP TIME: 15 MINUTES

WRAPS

1 medium jicama or turnip, peeled

1 avocado, sliced

1 large carrot, shredded or julienned

Several sprigs of fresh mint, chopped

DIPPING SAUCE*

2 tablespoons (28 ml) coconut aminos

2 teaspoons brown rice vinegar

(Optional) 1 teaspoon grated ginger

Slice the jicama or turnip thinly and carefully using a mandoline. Fill with the desired amount of avocado, carrot, and mint. Dip and enjoy!

*Alternatively, you could use Sweet and Spicy No Peanut Dipping Sauce (page 168).

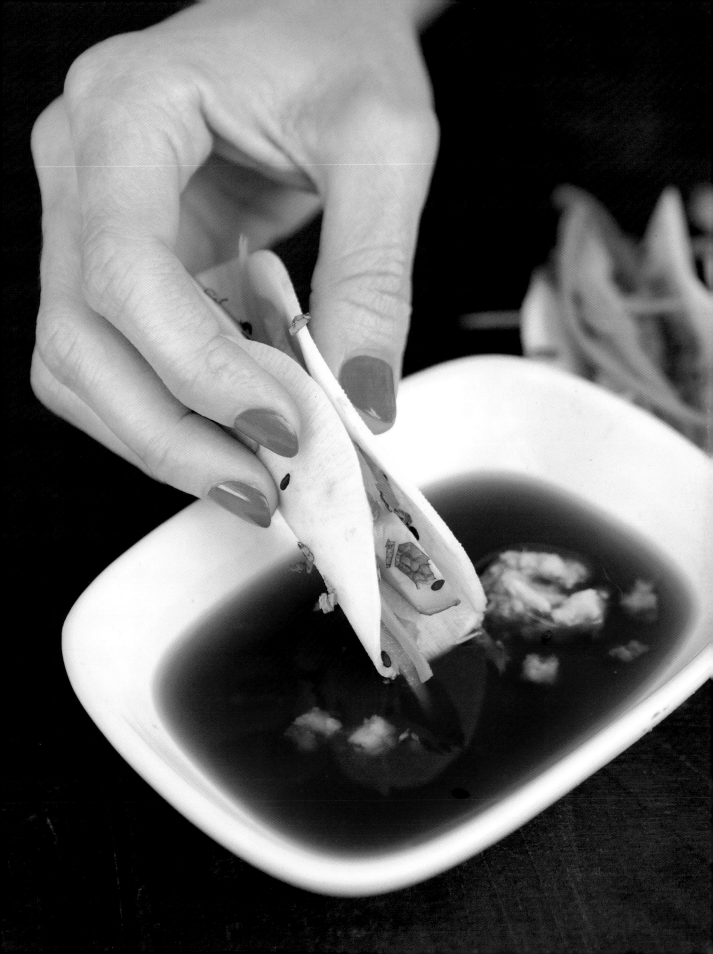

ALMOND-CRUSTED SALMON FILET (COOKED)

This is a nice addition to your Lunch Feast if you want to include a bit of protein in your cleanse. You can use store-bought almond meal or make your own by pulsing almonds in a food processor. Make it coarse or fine—either way is delicious.

MAKES 1 SERVING
PREP TIME: 10 MINUTES PLUS 10 TO 12 MINUTES TO BAKE

¼ pound (115 g) salmon filet

2 tablespoons (14 g) almond meal

⅛ teaspoon smoked paprika

⅛ teaspoon Italian seasoning

⅛ teaspoon onion powder

⅛ teaspoon sea salt

Dash of fresh pepper

1 teaspoon coconut oil, warmed to liquid

Wedge of lemon

Preheat oven to 425°F (220°C, or gas mark 7).

Rinse and pat dry the salmon filet and place, skin side down, in a baking dish or baking sheet lined with parchment paper.

Combine all the dry ingredients in a small bowl.

Drizzle the coconut oil over the filet and then sprinkle or dredge with the dry ingredients until well coated.

Bake for about 10 minutes or until desired the tenderness and serve with a lemon wedge.

CHEF TIP:

You could also use almond pulp left over from making milk. The pulp should be dried first, either by dehydrating it or baking it in the oven. Lay the pulp on a baking sheet lined with parchment paper and dry at the lowest setting for about twenty minutes or until dry. Grind in a food processor and it's ready to go.

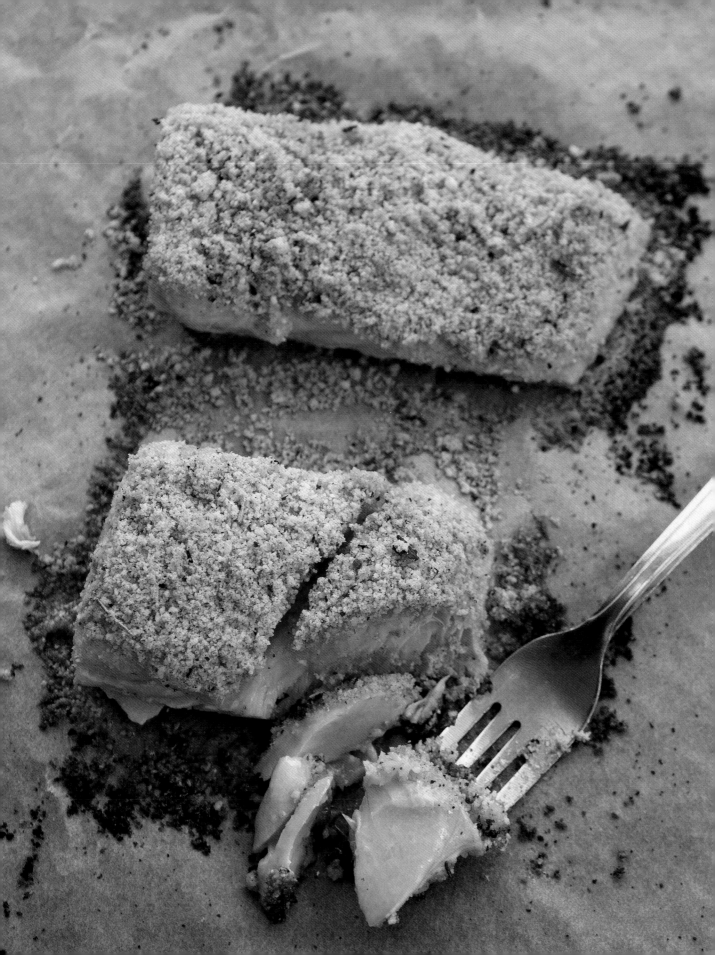

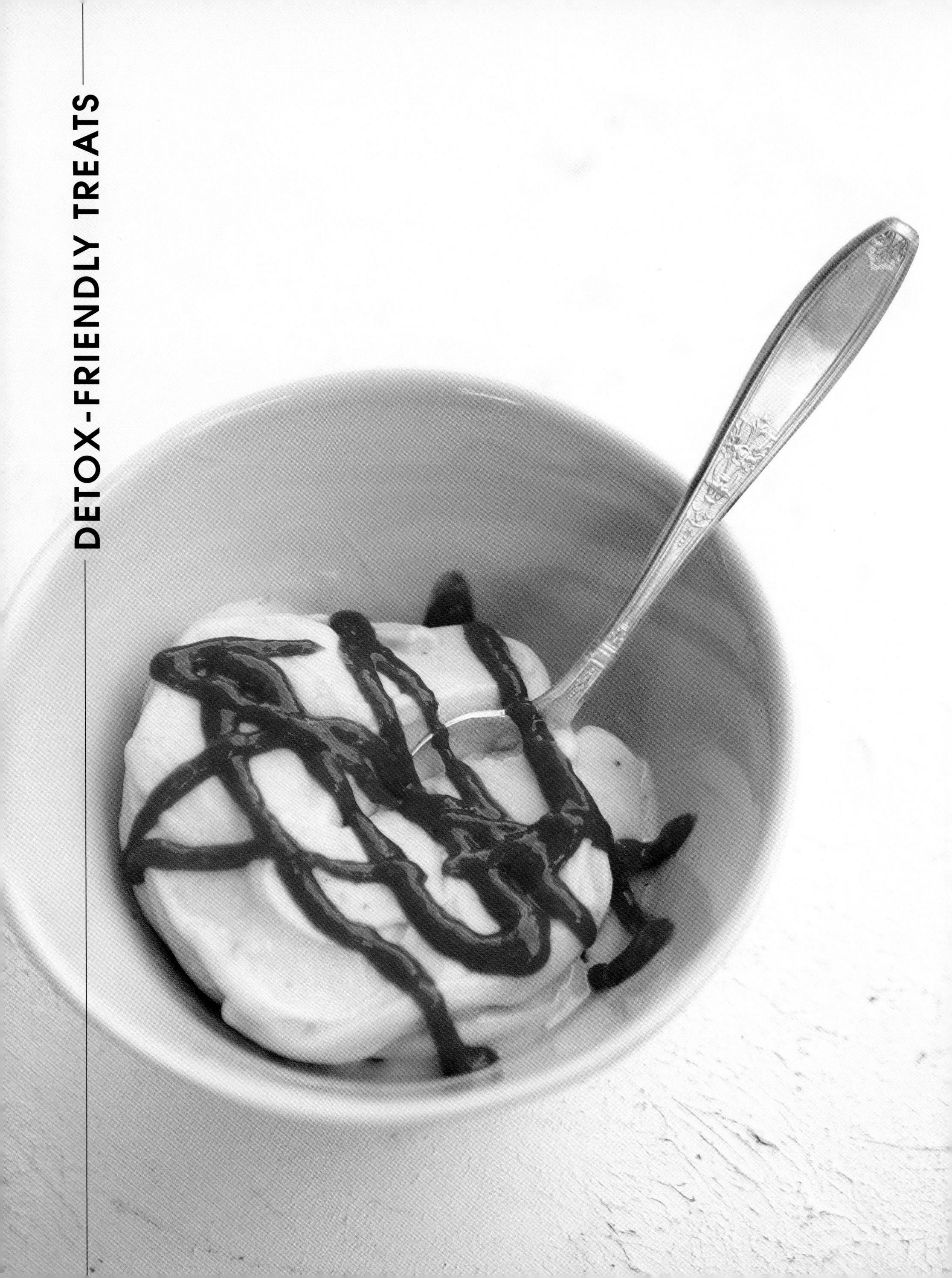

BANANA SOFT SERVE WITH RASPBERRY SAUCE

This is probably the most popular and easiest of all raw food desserts to make, but for the best results, you should use a masticating-type juicer with a blank screen (not the juicing screen) or a high-power blender with a tamper. A food processor works, but you won't get the same creamy texture. If you want to kick the wow factor up a notch, top it with melted Almond Butter Chocolate Bark (page 158).

MAKES 2 SERVINGS
PREP TIME: 15 MINUTES
PLAN AHEAD: FREEZE AT LEAST 2 CUPS (300 G) OF SLICED BANANAS.

2 cups (300 g) or more frozen banana chunks

RASPBERRY SAUCE

1 package (10 to 12 ounces [280 to 340 g]) frozen raspberries, thawed

2 tablespoons (28 g) coconut nectar or few drops of liquid stevia

FOR THE SAUCE

Process all the ingredients in blender or food processor until smooth.

FOR THE SOFT SERVE

Run the frozen banana pieces through your juicer using the blank plate. Transfer to serving bowls and pour the raspberry sauce over the bananas and enjoy. You can also add some chopped nuts or cacao nibs for some crunch.

HIGH SPEED BLENDER METHOD

Blend the frozen banana pieces using the tamper to push pieces into the blades. Use more banana if needed. Blend just until smooth.

FOOD PROCESSOR METHOD

Purée in a food processor for about 5 minutes, scraping down the sides as needed.

NOTE: There are also gadgets that are made specifically for these types of frozen desserts like the Yonanas Maker.

CHEF TIP:
You can skip the raspberry sauce and just push the frozen raspberries and bananas through the juicer together.

CHOCOLATE CHIA SILK

Here's a way to get your chocolate mousse fix without throwing your detox efforts out the window. This is thicker than regular chia pudding because the coconut fat and lecithin form a mousse-like texture that is to live for. This doesn't work as well with store-bought coconut milk beverage as it is too low fat to create a silky texture.

MAKES 2 SERVINGS
PREP TIME: 10 MINUTES PLUS 4 TO 6 HOURS TO CHILL
PLAN AHEAD: YOU WILL NEED 1 CUP (235 ML) COCONUT MILK (PAGE 72).

CHIA SILK

1 cup (235 ml) Coconut Milk (page 72)

2 tablespoons (11 g) cacao powder

2 tablespoons (24 g) xylitol granules*

Few drops of liquid stevia, to taste*

2 tablespoons (16 g) lecithin powder or granules

Dash of vanilla powder or ½ teaspoon vanilla extract

¼ cup (52 g) chia seeds

OPTIONAL TOPPINGS

Cacao nibs

Chopped nuts

Bananas

Berries

Process the coconut milk, cacao powder, sweeteners, lecithin, and vanilla in a blender. Transfer to a small bowl and add the chia seeds. Mix well and allow to sit for 5 to 10 minutes. Stir again to remove any lumps and then pour into two individual ramekins or small mason jars. Place in the refrigerator for 4 to 6 hours or until all the liquid is absorbed and begins to set.

Top with cacao nibs, chopped nuts, bananas, or berries if desired.

*For this low-glycemic dessert, I like to use both xylitol and stevia. You can substitute with another sweetener if you prefer.

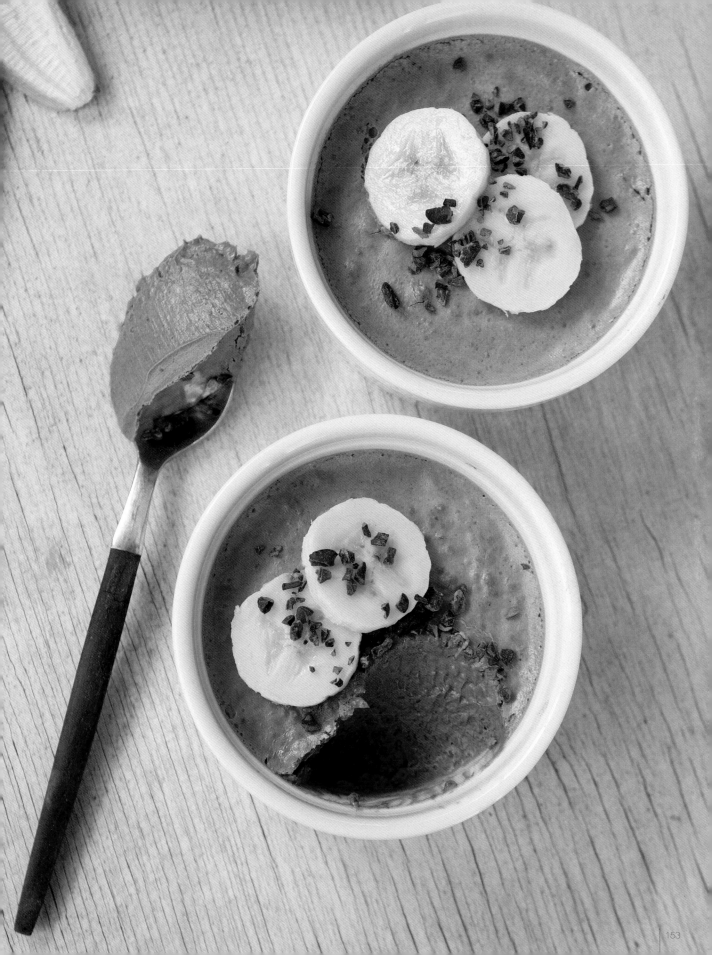

TROPICAL BLISS PUDDING

This is fruit pudding you'll dream about. Enjoy it for breakfast or dessert.

MAKES 1 TO 2 SERVINGS
PREP TIME: 5 MINUTES

2 cups (280 g) cubed papaya

1 ripe banana, peeled

1 tablespoon (15 g) raw tahini

¼ teaspoon cinnamon

Liquid stevia or your favorite sweetener, to taste

1 tablespoon (5 g) shredded coconut

1 tablespoon (8 g) cacao nibs

Place all the ingredients except for the coconut and cacao nibs in a food processor and blend until smooth. Pour into a small bowl and top with the coconut and cacao nibs.

HEALTH NOTE:

Most store-bought tahini contains roasted sesame seeds, so look for a raw brand that uses sprouted sesame seeds to get the most nutrients. My favorite brand is from Living Tree Community Foods. Sesame seeds are rich in minerals like calcium and iron, B vitamins, protein, and they're a good source of the amino acid methionine, which aids in liver detoxification. If you want to get more tahini in your diet, try the Beanless Spinach Hummus on page 165 or Garlic Tahini Dressing on page 127.

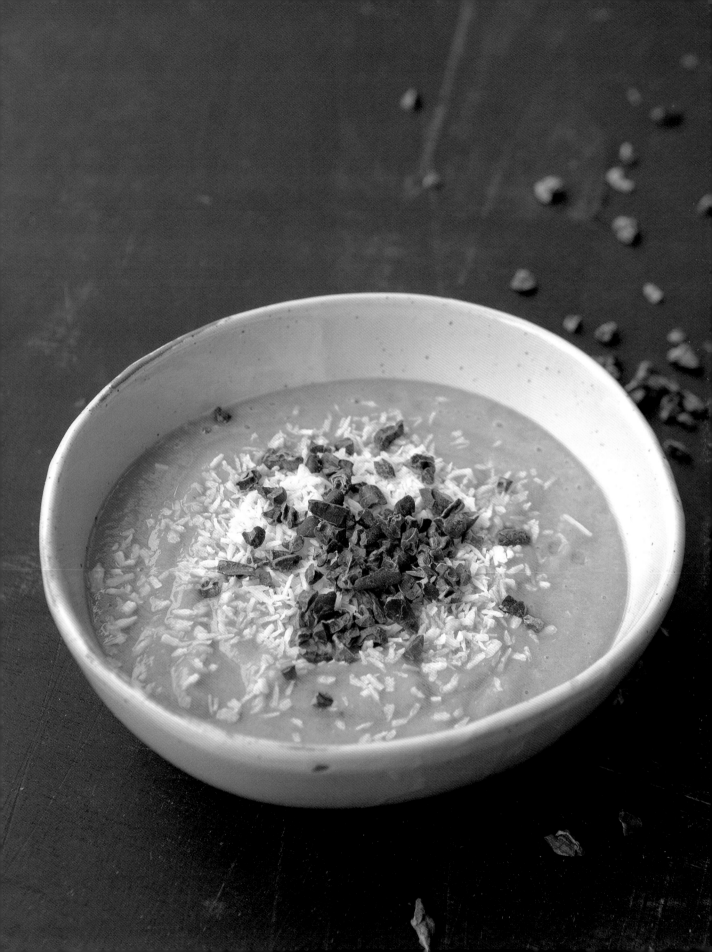

COCONUT-BASIL SORBET

Rich, creamy, and low-glycemic—that's what I look for in a dessert. This is a great summertime treat you can make instantly in your high-power blender. And if sweet basil isn't your thing, replace with fresh mint or omit it altogether.

MAKES 4 SERVINGS
PREP TIME: 15 MINUTES

1 cup (80 g) young Thai coconut meat

½ of a lemon, peeled, seeded

½ of a lime, peeled

¼ cup (10 g) loosely packed fresh basil leaves

3 cups (420 g) ice cubes (if using a high speed blender)

   or 1 cup (235 ml) water (if using a conventional blender)

Several drops of liquid stevia, xylitol granules, or your favorite sweetener

IF USING A HIGH SPEED BLENDER:

Blend the coconut, lemon, lime, basil, and sweetener. Add more sweetener after blended if needed, as it will get diluted once you add ice. (I err on the side of more sweetness.)

Add the ice and blend using the tamper to push ingredients into the blades. Continue until smooth but still icy. Do not overblend. You can place your container in the freezer for a few minutes to firm up if it's too runny.

NOTE: You will have better results using a 4-cup (1 L) container as opposed to an 8-cup (2 L) one. If you only have a large container, then double the recipe or follow the conventional blender method.

IF USING A CONVENTIONAL BLENDER:

Replace the ice with 1 cup (235 ml) water and blend until smooth. Process in an ice cream maker according to manufacturer's instructions.

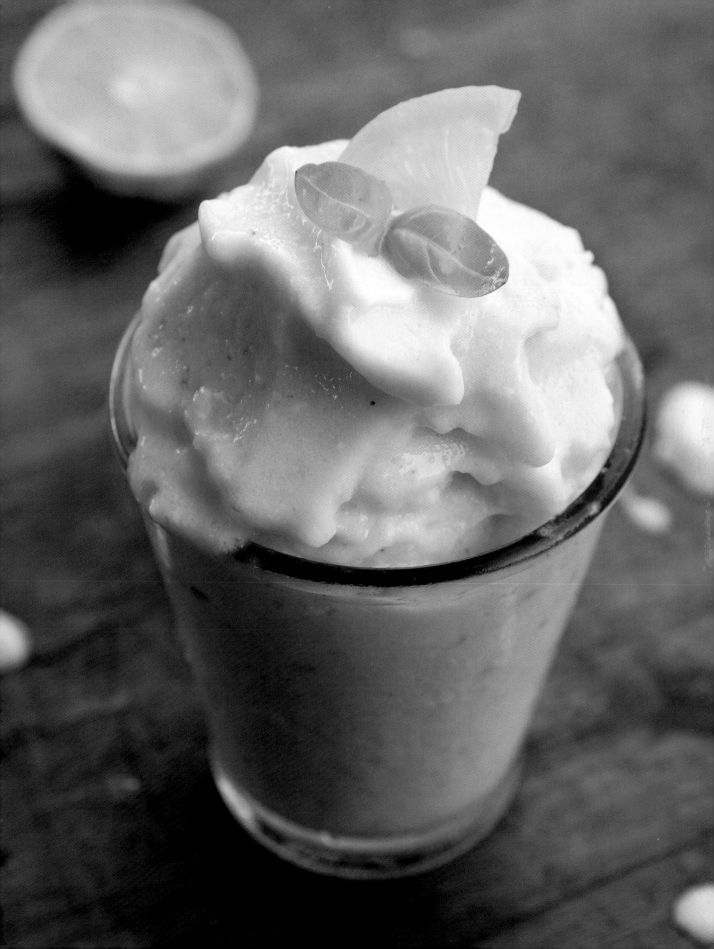

ALMOND BUTTER CHOCOLATE BARK

Cleansing is hard, so I believe sometimes you need a little reward to keep going. Just promise me you won't go overboard and eat the whole batch at once. This melt-in-your-mouth (and sometimes your hand) chocolate is too good to be true. I sweeten it with xylitol and stevia to make it low glycemic and completely guilt free. If you're cutting out all sugar, skip the goji berries, as well. For those who don't like xylitol and stevia, you could use coconut palm sugar instead.

MAKES 12 SERVINGS
PREP TIME: 15 MINUTES

ALMOND BUTTER CHOCOLATE BARK

⅓ cup (75 g) coconut oil, warmed to liquid

⅔ cup (60 g) cacao powder

¼ cup (65 g) raw almond butter

1½ tablespoons (18 g) xylitol granules

Liquid stevia, to taste

Dash of vanilla powder

3 tablespoons (24 g) or more cacao nibs

3 tablespoons (17 g) or more goji berries

Pinch of sea salt

OPTIONAL ADD-INS

Reishi powder

Chaga powder

Ashwagandha powder

Maca powder

Blend the coconut oil, cacao powder, almond butter, xylitol, stevia, and vanilla in a blender until smooth. Add more sweetener if desired. You can also add a small amount of powdered reishi, chaga, ashwaganda, maca, or any other superfoods at this time. Go easy, as your chocolate could start to get bitter.

Pour the chocolate over a small baking sheet lined with parchment or wax paper. Sprinkle with cacao nibs, goji berries, and sea salt.

Chill in the freezer for 15 minutes or until solid. Break into desired size pieces by hand. Store in a container in the refrigerator or freezer.

CHEF TIP:

You can use the mixture as a dip or topping by pouring it into a small bowl or squeeze bottle. Use it as a fondue for strawberries, bananas, or whatever else your heart desires. It's also an awesome topping for Banana Soft Serve (page 151).

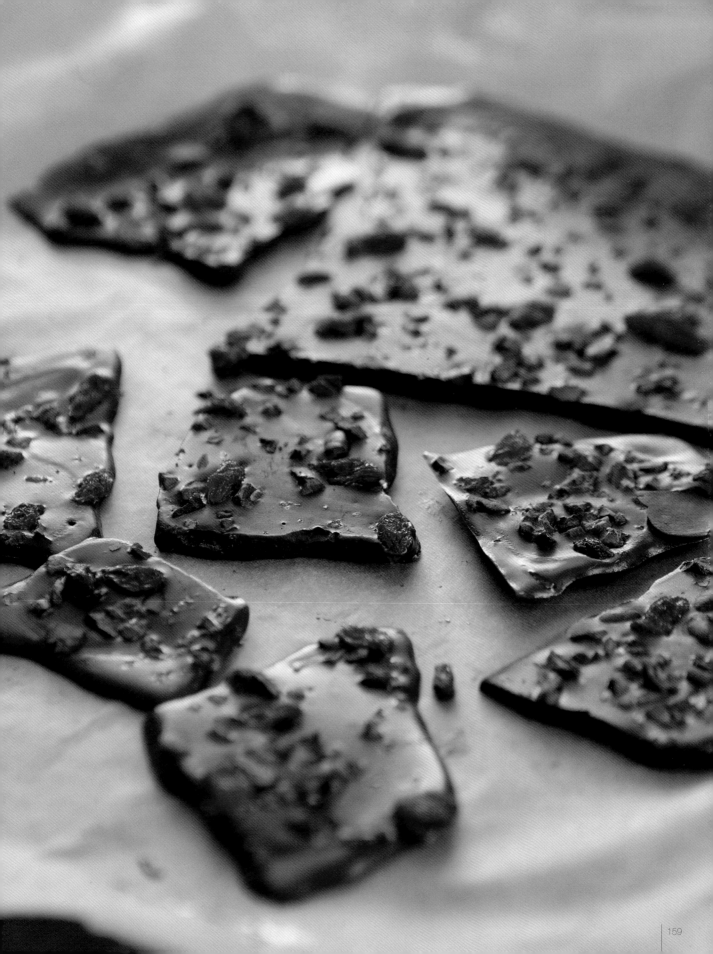

FROZEN FRUIT YOGURT

These fruity frozen yogurts are crazy good and make a cooling treat on a hot summer day. They work best using the coconut yogurt recipe from this book. The fat content gives it amazing creaminess and body. If you're in a pinch or just prefer a lighter treat, you can use store-bought coconut yogurt. If it gets too thin, chill it briefly before serving, pour it into ice pop trays, or churn it in an ice cream maker according to the manufacturer's instructions.

MAKES 3 TO 4 SERVINGS
PREP TIME: 5 MINUTES
PLAN AHEAD: YOU WILL NEED 1 CUP (230 G) COCONUT YOGURT (PAGE 168).

SPICED PEACHES

1 cup (230 g) Coconut Yogurt (page 168)

2 cups (500 g) frozen sliced peaches

1 teaspoon grated ginger

1 teaspoon lemon zest

Few drops of liquid stevia

STRAWBERRY BASIL

1 cup (230 g) Coconut Yogurt (page 168)

2 cups (510 g) frozen strawberries

2 small basil leaves

Few drops of liquid stevia

MANGO LASSI

1 cup (230 g) Coconut Yogurt (page 168)

2 cups (330 g) frozen mango chunks

¼ teaspoon garam masala or cardamom

Few drops of liquid stevia

Blend all the ingredients for the desired flavor for about 1 minute or until creamy, using the tamper the entire time to keep things moving. Do not overblend.

NOTE: This recipe works best in a high-speed blender with a tamper. If you don't have a power blender, use fresh or thawed fruit and blend into a smoothie consistency. Pour into an ice cream maker and follow manufacturer's instructions or pour into ice pop molds.

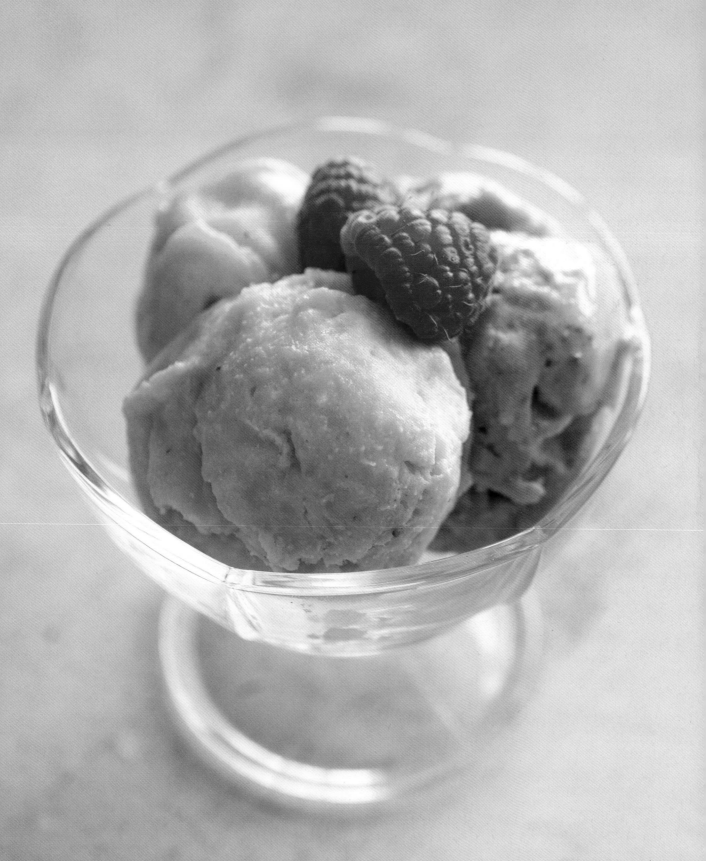

FIESTA FRUIT CUPS

This fun and colorful fruit salad in a cup couldn't be easier to make. The lime and cayenne compliment the tropical flavors, while the jicama gives it some crunch.

PREP TIME: 10 MINUTES

FRUIT

Jicama spears

Watermelon spears

Papaya spears

Pineapple spears

Mango wedges

TOPPING

1 lime, cut into wedges

Cayenne pepper

Arrange any combination of the fruit spears in a short cup or glass and top with a squeeze of lime and a dash of cayenne pepper.

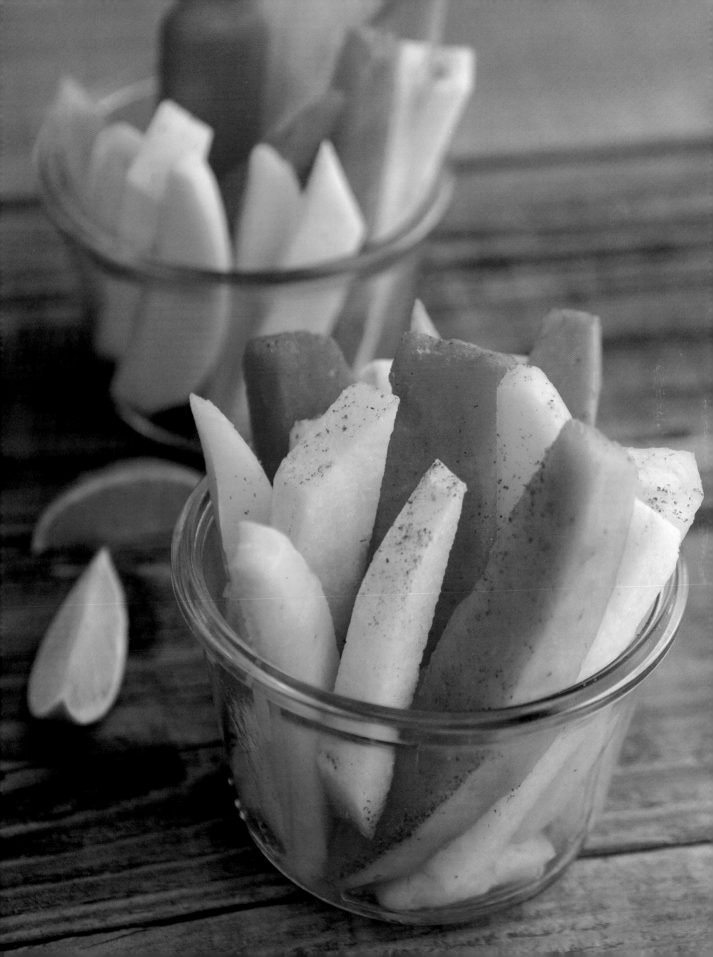

DIPS, SAUCES, AND SPREADS

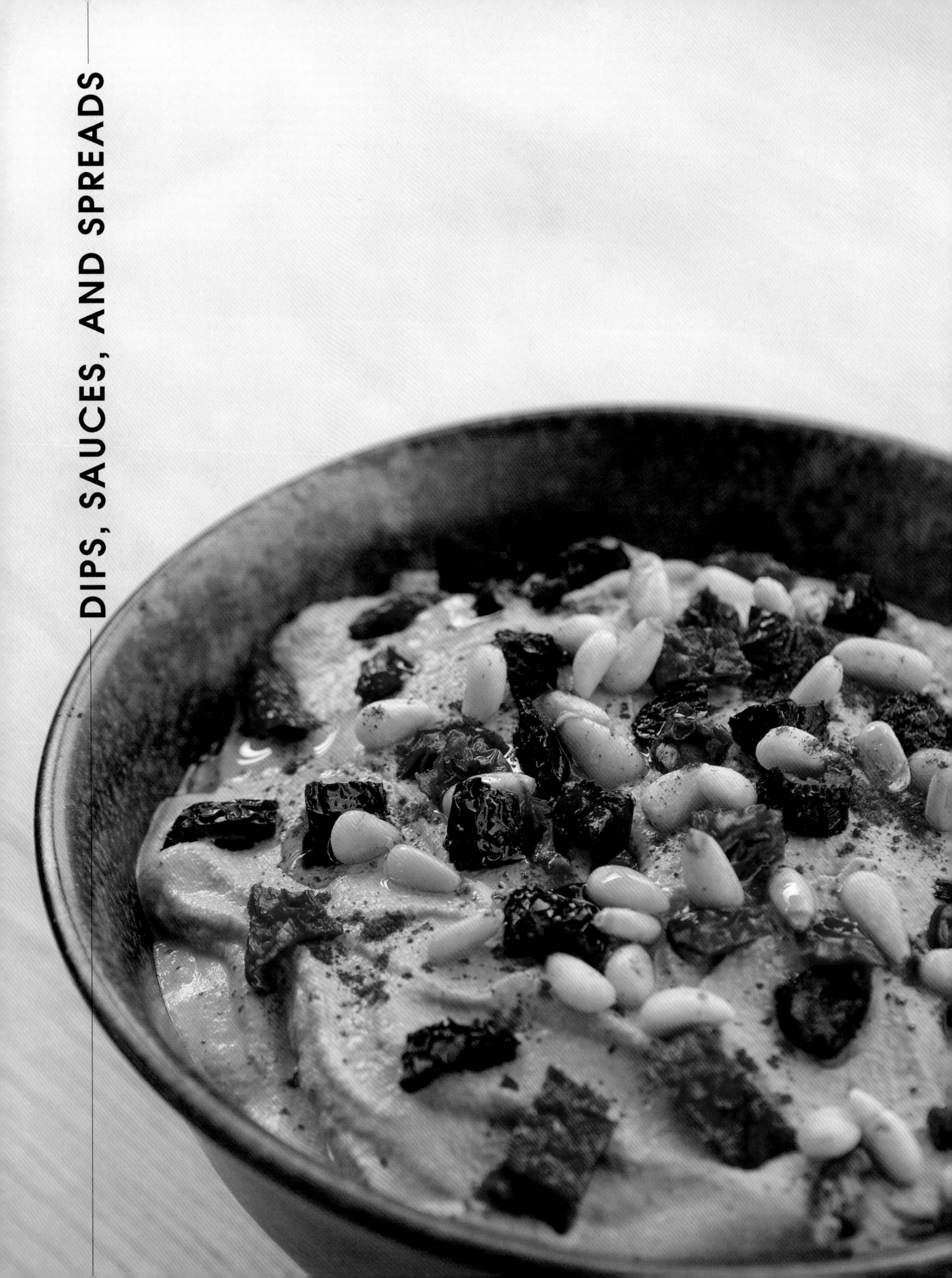

BEANLESS SPINACH HUMMUS

This makes a great dip for crudités or raw crackers, or use it as a spread for raw wraps like the Green Submarine Wrap (page 138). If you don't have a high-speed blender with a tamper, use a food processor.

MAKES 4 SERVINGS
PREP TIME: 15 MINUTES

1 cup (120 g) chopped zucchini

1 cup (30 g) spinach

½ cup (120 g) raw tahini

¼ cup (60 ml) lemon juice

2 tablespoons (15 g) hemp seeds

1 clove of garlic

1 tablespoon (15 ml) olive oil

½ teaspoon cumin

½ teaspoon paprika

¼ teaspoon sea salt

Dash of cayenne pepper

OPTIONAL TOPPINGS

Botija olives

Raw pine nuts

Paprika

Olive oil

Sun-dried tomatoes

Process all the ingredients in a blender or food processor until smooth. Adjust seasonings to taste.

Transfer the mixture to a small serving bowl and add the desired toppings. Chill to firm.

POWER PESTO SPREAD

This power-packed, cheesy pesto spread can be used in wraps or smothered over a raw cracker or celery stick.

MAKES 4 SERVINGS
PREP TIME: 15 MINUTES
PLAN AHEAD: SOAK ½ CUP (68 G) RAW PINE NUTS AND ½ CUP (70 G) RAW CASHEWS FOR 2 HOURS AND THEN DRAIN AND RINSE.

½ cup (68 g) raw pine nuts, soaked 2 hours

½ cup (70 g) raw cashews, soaked 2 hours

2 tablespoons (15 g) hemp seeds

¼ teaspoon sea salt

1 cup (40 g) basil, packed

½ cup (8 g) cilantro, packed

½ cup (10 g) arugula, packed

2 tablespoons (28 ml) olive oil

2 cloves of garlic, crushed

(Optional) ⅛ teaspoon spirulina powder

In a food processor, blend the pine nuts, cashews, hemp seeds, and sea salt until it becomes a creamy paste. Scrape down the sides as needed. Transfer to a small bowl.

Add the basil, cilantro, arugula, olive oil, garlic, and spirulina to food processor and blend well, scraping down the sides as needed. Transfer to the bowl with the nut mixture and mix by hand until combined.

PESTO SAUCE

This sauce is aromatic and bursting with flavor. Try tossing it with zucchini noodles for a satisfying meal that will have you dreaming of Italy.

MAKES ENOUGH SAUCE FOR 6 MEDIUM SPIRALIZED ZUCCHINIS
PREP TIME: 10 MINUTES

2 cups (80 g) basil leaves, packed

¼ cup (60 ml) olive oil

3 to 4 cloves of garlic, crushed

½ teaspoon sea salt

½ cup (60 g) hemp seeds or (68 g) raw pine nuts

Place all the ingredients except for the hemp seeds (or pine nuts) in a food processor and blend until smooth. Add the hemp seeds and pulse a few times until incorporated.

TOMATO MARINARA

Deliciously fresh and just as flavorful as your grandma's traditional red sauce. Toss with zucchini noodles for a pasta dish that won't make you sleepy.

MAKES ENOUGH SAUCE FOR 6 MEDIUM SPIRALIZED ZUCCHINIS
PREP TIME: 15 MINUTES

½ of a red bell pepper, seeded and chopped

2 tablespoons (130 g) sun-dried tomato powder*

1 to 2 tablespoons (15 to 28 ml) olive oil

2 tablespoons (3 g) fresh basil or 1 teaspoon dried

1 tablespoon (4 g) fresh oregano or 1 teaspoon dried

½ of a Medjool date

2 cloves of garlic

½ teaspoon sea salt, or to taste

¼ teaspoon crushed red pepper

3 cups (540 g) chopped tomatoes

Blend all the ingredients except for the tomatoes in a food processor until smooth. Add the tomatoes and pulse until incorporated but still a little chunky.

Toss with the zucchini noodles or ribbons and garnish with raw pine nuts, olives, and/or diced bell peppers.

*Make sun-dried tomato powder by grinding sun-dried tomatoes in a spice grinder. Alternatively, you can use a few pieces of oil-packed sun-dried tomatoes.

PARMESAN "CHEESE"

This is a great topping for all the Italian dishes in this book. You can even sprinkle it over salads and soups for a little salty, cheesy goodness.

MAKES 8 SERVINGS
PREP TIME: 5 MINUTES

1 cup (140 g) raw cashews, not soaked

1 clove of garlic, crushed

½ tablespoon nutritional yeast

¼ teaspoon sea salt

Pulse all the ingredients in a food processor until the mixture becomes the texture of parmesan cheese. Store in an airtight jar in the refrigerator.

COCONUT YOGURT

Add this to smoothies for richness and a boost of beneficial bacteria or put a dollop over fresh fruit. For a time-saving shortcut, check the freezer section at your health food store for the brand Exotic Superfoods, which sells bags and bottles of organic young Thai coconut meat and water that are ready to use.

MAKES ABOUT 3 CUPS (690 G)
PREP TIME: 10 MINUTES PLUS FERMENTATION TIME

2 cups (160 g) young Thai coconut meat (about 3 coconuts)

⅔ cup (160 ml) coconut water

2 probiotic capsules or ½ of a packet of kefir starter

Blend the coconut meat and coconut water until completely smooth. Add the probiotics and blend briefly. Transfer to a glass container with a lid and allow it to ferment at room temperature for 4 to 12 hours. The longer it sits and the warmer the environment, the more tart it will taste and the more fermented it will be. If you ferment for too long, it will actually become effervescent and sour.

Store in the refrigerator for up to 7 days. I like to divide my yogurt into ½-pint (235 ml) mason jars, freeze them, and thaw a jar out as needed. They can last several weeks in the freezer without diminishing much of the probiotic effects.

SWEET AND SPICY NO PEANUT DIPPING SAUCE

This is the next best thing to actual Thai peanut sauce, but without the aflatoxin, a toxic mold and known carcinogen found in moldy peanuts. This sauce is awesome with the Asian Root Wraps (page 146) and Ginger-Miso Veggie Rolls (page 136).

MAKES 4 SERVINGS
PREP TIME: 10 MINUTES

½ cup (130 g) raw almond butter

¼ cup (60 ml) water

3 tablespoons (45 ml) coconut aminos

1 tablespoon (15 ml) brown rice vinegar

1 tablespoon (14 g) coconut nectar

½ tablespoon grated ginger

1 clove of garlic, crushed

¼ teaspoon crushed red pepper

Use a mini blender or hand-whisk to blend all the ingredients until smooth.

QUEEN OF GREEN DIP

This green bowl of deliciousness is a cross between guacamole and spinach dip. For a quick snack, stuff mushroom caps with it or use it as a dip or spread like in Green Submarine Wraps (page 138).

MAKES 2 TO 3 SERVINGS
PREP TIME: 15 MINUTES

1 large avocado

½ cup (30 g) spinach, finely chopped

1 leaf kale, destemmed and finely chopped

½ tomato, diced

¼ cup (4 g) cilantro, finely chopped

2 tablespoons (20 g) red onion

1 small clove of garlic, crushed

½ of a jalapeno, seeded

Juice from ½ of a lime

Sea salt, to taste

In a small bowl, combine all ingredients. I like it chunky; if you prefer it smoother or want to save time, place all ingredients except tomato and red onion in a food processor and blend until smooth. Transfer to a bowl and stir in tomato and onion.

QUICK PICKLED CABBAGE

This is a great little condiment to put in the Green Submarine Wraps (page 138) or Ginger-Miso Veggie Rolls (page 136), or thrown into a salad for a little zing and a splash of color.

MAKES 8 SERVINGS
PREP TIME: 5 MINUTES, PLUS 1 TO 6 HOURS TO MARINATE

¼ cup (60 ml) apple cider vinegar

½ tablespoon coconut nectar

Pinch of sea salt

Combine all the ingredients in a bowl. Place a plate or bowl with a weight (like a mason jar of water) on top of the mixture and allow it to sit for 1 to 6 hours. It will soften and release more liquid the longer you let it sit.

The cabbage will keep for 5 days in the refrigerator.

Glossary

ashwagandha:

Used traditionally in Ayurvedic medicine, this adaptogenic herb is useful for helping to relieve stress and anxiety and supporting adrenal and brain function.

bee pollen:

This is considered to be a superfood among athletes. It is very good source of complete protein and high in B vitamins, phytonutrients, and enzymes.

blue-green algae:

This is a type of microalgae that contains an array of vitamins, minerals, enzymes, phytonutrients, and amino acids and is high in chlorophyll. It is a popular superfood used in smoothies and salads.

Bragg Apple Cider Vinegar:

This is a raw vinegar that works great in dressings and sauces and can be taken with water as a digestive aid.

burdock root:

Also called gogo, this tuber is a tasty vegetable that has been used medicinally for centuries in Asian cultures. It's a very powerful blood cleanser, diuretic, detoxifier, and skin healer.

cacao butter:

This is the fat that has been separated from the cacao bean. It is used for making chocolate and other desserts.

cacao powder:

This is ground cacao beans, also known as cocoa powder. Most supermarkets carry only heated cacao, so find a reputable raw brand at a health food store or online. It's the best plant source of magnesium and a great source of amino acids, especially tryptophan, which helps create serotonin and also contains the stimulating alkaloid theobromine.

camu camu:

This is a superfood from South America made from the berries of the camu camu bush. It is considered to have the highest vitamin C content of any plant.

carob powder:

This comes from the carob pods of the carob tree. It looks much like cacao, but without the stimulating effects or bitterness. It is sweet and can be used as a substitute for cacao in desserts and smoothies.

Celtic sea salt:

This is a moist, sun-dried sea salt that contains an array of trace minerals.

chaga:

This is a medicinal mushroom that contains powerful immune system boosters and anticancer properties. It's considered a superfood for its extremely high ORAC value (ORAC stands for oxygen radical absorbance capacity—the method to measure antioxidant content) and an adaptogen for its ability to strengthen the adrenals and body in times of stress.

chia seeds:

Ancient food of the Aztecs, this gluten-free seed is high in essential fatty acids, complete protein, and fiber.

coconut nectar:

This is a sap similar to maple syrup that comes from palm trees. It has a molasses type flavor and a high mineral content.

dulse:

This is a mild-tasting seaweed that you can buy as little flakes or as larger strips. No soaking is necessary, and it can be eaten straight out of the bag. I like storing the flakes in a sugar dispenser to make it easy to sprinkle on salads.

goji berries:

These are rich red-orange berries high in antioxidants that have been used for centuries in Chinese medicine as a powerful tonic herb.

Himalayan pink salt:

This is a prized, high-mineral salt excavated from the Himalayan mountains.

jicama:

This is a sweet and crunchy root vegetable from Mexico similar to a potato that can be enjoyed raw.

kelp granules:

These make a great salt substitute or are useful if you want to give something a fishy taste, such as in a Thai sauce or "tuna" salad.

kelp noodles:

A sea vegetable product resembling glass noodles, they take on the flavor of whatever sauce you use them with. Rinse them well before eating.

kombu:

This is a type of kelp that is very high in natural iodine and very delicious in vegetable stock and soups.

lecithin:

This is a powder usually made from soy that is useful as an emulsifier and thickener in recipes. Look for sunflower lecithin powder or granules or a non-GMO soy lecithin powder. It is also a good source of choline.

maca:

This is a Peruvian root that is dried and ground into a flour. Known as an adaptogenic superfood, it helps support the hormonal, nervous, and cardiovascular systems.

Medjool dates:

These are soft and chewy dates that have a lovely caramel-type flavor and a higher water content than other varieties.

methylsulfonylmethane (MSM):

This is a naturally occurring sulfur compound that is effective at lowering inflammation, like arthritis, in the body. It can be added to beverages and smoothies.

miso:

This is a fermented Asian condiment usually made from soybeans and rice. I use chickpea miso paste from Miso Master because it is soy-free and has a very nice, mild flavor.

nori:

This is the most popular species of seaweed and is used for making sushi rolls. All nori sheets are toasted unless marked otherwise.

nutritional yeast:

This is a food supplement that is high in B vitamins and that gives raw food dishes a cheesy flavor, similar to that of Parmesan cheese.

palm sugar:

This is an unrefined sweetener made from the sap of coconut trees. It has a brown sugar–like flavor, is high in minerals, and can be used in place of xylitol or evaporated cane juice.

raw tahini:

This is a delicious paste made of sesame seeds. It's also a good source of plant based calcium. Most brands of tahini are roasted, so check the label.

spirulina:

This is an ancient single-celled blue-green algae high in protein, vitamins, minerals, enzymes, phytonutrients, and chlorophyll.

stevia:

The leaves of the stevia plant have been used as a sweetener for centuries. It's extremely sweet with a bitter, licorice aftertaste. It's an acquired taste, but favorable for those who are avoiding sugar. I use a liquid unreconstituted stevia from Omica Organics in my beverages and smoothies.

superfoods:

These are foods that have a very high ORAC value as well as other qualities that are extraordinary. They're considered to be more like whole food supplements.

tamari:

This is a fermented and gluten-free soy sauce appropriate for people with wheat allergies.

xylitol:

This is a low-glycemic sweetener usually made from birch trees and corn. It looks and tastes very much like white sugar but without the blood-spiking qualities. It's a safe alternative sweetener for diabetics, cancer patients, or anyone following a low-sugar diet.

Index

RESOURCES

INGREDIENTS AND EQUIPMENT
Judita Wignall, www.juditawignall.com
City & Sea Trading, www.cityandseatrading.com
Living Light Marketplace, shop.rawfoodchef.com
The Raw Food World, www.therawfoodworld.com
Vita-Mix Blenders, www.vitamix.com
Stormy Monday Denim & Goods, www.stormymondaygoods.com
Zoe Ceramics, www.zoeceramics.com

RAW AND PLANT-BASED LIFESTYLE WEBSITES
Cleanse America, www.cleanseamerica.com
Upgrade Your Plate, www.upgradeyourplate.com
Vibrant Living with Dr. Ritamarie, www.drritamarie.com

RAW FOOD AND HEALTH BLOGS
City & Sea Living, cityandsealiving.blogspot.com
Choosing Raw, www.choosingraw.com
Raw on $10 a Day (or Less!), www.rawon10.blogspot.com
Rawmazing, www.rawmazing.com
Oh She Glows, www.ohsheglows.com

RAW FOOD CULINARY PROGRAMS
Living Light Culinary Institute, www.rawfoodchef.com
Matthew Kenny Cuisine, www.matthewkenneycuisine.com

BECOME A CERTIFIED HEALTH COACH
Institute for Integrative Nutrition, www.integrativenutrition.com
Tell them I sent you or email me for more info.

ACKNOWLEDGMENTS

I am so grateful for everyone at Quarry Books for giving me another opportunity to share my recipes and for supporting me the past few years. Thank you Winnie, Tiffany, Renae, and David for allowing me to pursue my vision for this project.

Much love to my artistic team: Peilin Breller for her superb styling, and my husband extraordinaire, Matt Wignall, for photographing my recipes so beautifully, and Amy Sterner for her invaluable assistance. Special thanks to Britney Cherry for assistance, set design, and the downtown LA photo (pages 10 and 11), and Noah Rodriguez and Tyler Day for the graphic design assistance.

Thank you to Vitamix for making the best blender ever and for supporting my work the past few years. Thanks also to Stormy Monday Goods for making me their culinary team rider and blessing me with their gorgeous handcrafted boards. Thank you also to Zoe Gardner for your amazing ceramic work for this book. Thanks to Alex and Mary at www.maryscostarica.com for photo locations and a healthy place to write and unwind!

Thank you to my star recipe testers Anita Repp, Bradford Peter, and Sandra Andrea Schneider and most of all thank you to my readers for inpiring and bringing out the best in me.

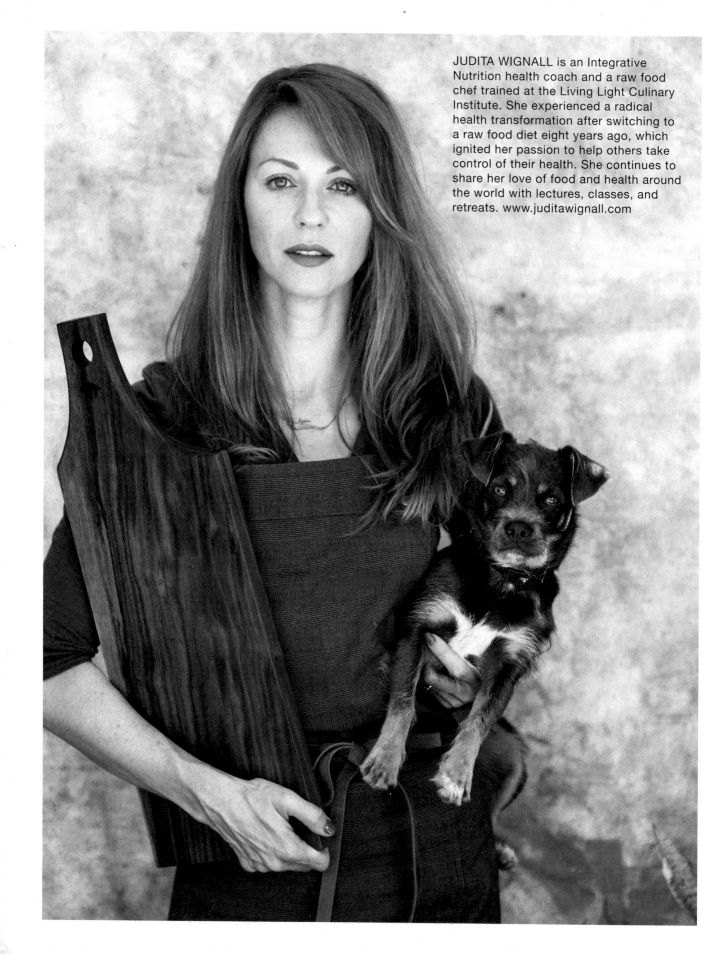

JUDITA WIGNALL is an Integrative Nutrition health coach and a raw food chef trained at the Living Light Culinary Institute. She experienced a radical health transformation after switching to a raw food diet eight years ago, which ignited her passion to help others take control of their health. She continues to share her love of food and health around the world with lectures, classes, and retreats. www.juditawignall.com